Healing Emotions
WITH ESSENTIAL OIL

Rebecca Park Totilo

Healing Emotions With Essential Oil
Copyright © 2023 by Rebecca Park Totilo

All rights reserved. No part of this book may be reproduced or transmitted in any form or by any means without the author's written permission.

Printed in the United States of America.

Published by Rebecca at the Well Foundation.

No part of this publication may be reproduced, stored in a retrieval system or transmitted in any form by any means—electronic, mechanical, photocopy, recording, or otherwise—without written permission of the copyright holder, except as provided by USA copyright law.

Disclaimer Notice: The information contained in this book is intended for educational purposes only and is not meant to substitute for medical care or prescribe treatment for any specific health condition. Please see a qualified healthcare provider for medical treatment. The author and publisher assume no responsibility or liability for any person or group for any loss, damage, or injury resulting from using or misusing any information in this book. No express or implied guarantee is given regarding the effects of using any of the products described herein.

Paperback ISBN: 979-8-9872464-1-2
Electronic ISBN: 979-8-9872464-2-9

HI, I AM REBECCA

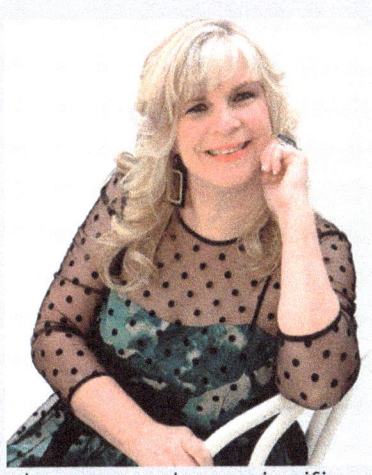

We all have one thing in common, regardless of age, lifestyle, or geographic location, and that is we all experience emotions every day. Emotions are an inescapable part of being human and can significantly impact our happiness and well-being. Although emotions are somewhat mysterious, they can be characterized as complex internal reactions that will differ from person to person.

Everyone has different personalities and life experiences, so it only makes sense that we would all deal with emotions differently. We all have different ways of responding to and processing emotions, and everyone expresses their feelings in individual ways.

While our emotions can impact our quality of life, we do know that they play a significant role in shaping our motivations. Our responses to feelings can improve or worsen our quality of life, depending on how we choose to respond based on our personality or experiences.

Uncontrolled emotions can negatively affect one's quality of life by harming their emotional or physical well-being. Conversely, experiencing positive emotions and finding healthy ways to deal with negative emotions can lead to an improved quality of life. Emotions are a universal experience, and we will never be able to escape them entirely. Whether we choose to deal with our unpleasant emotions or leave them unchecked is up to us.

In my own life, I have found essential oils to be a miracle in a small bottle. They transformed my health not only physically but emotionally. Shortly after discovering essential oils, I learned of their power to help me overcome the emotional issues that held me back. Through this life experience, I will share how you can release negative emotions by using oils instead of allowing them to rule you. With essential oils, you will learn how to relax your mind and body, allowing you to enjoy life more without the constant worry that stress brings.

I pray you will find peace and comfort in using essential oils for those moments when emotions try to get the best of you.

Peace,

Rebecca Park Totilo

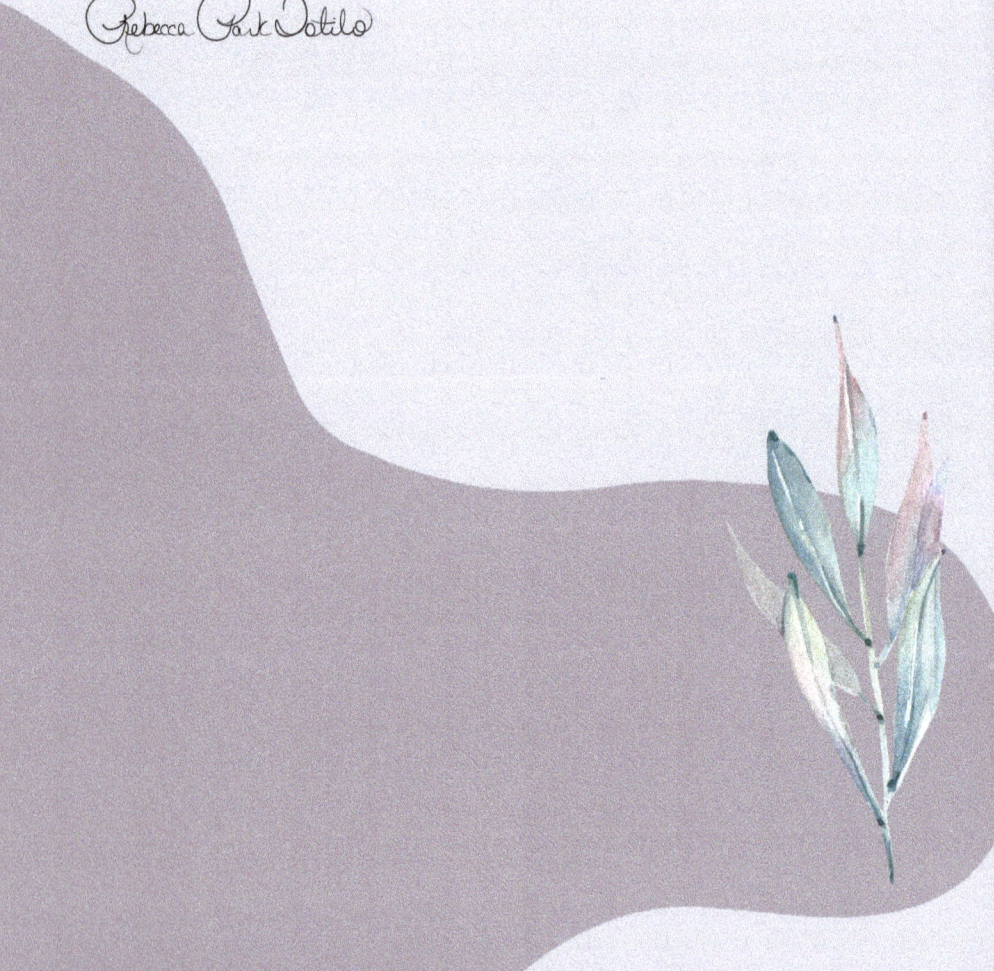

CONTENTS

INTRODUCTION TO EMOTIONAL HEALING　1

USING ESSENTIAL OILS TO SUPPORT YOUR
EMOTIONAL HEALTH　5

EMOTIONAL HEALING WITH OILS　11

WHY USE ESSENTIAL OILS FOR MOODS　15

THE SCIENTIFIC EVIDENCE BEHIND
AROMATHERAPY　19

GOVERNING YOUR EMOTIONAL
RESPONSE　33

ESSENTIAL OILS FOR EMOTIONS　39

COMMON EMOTIONS AND ESSENTIAL OILS	77
METHODS OF USE: AROMATICALLY	89
PERSONAL INHALERS	95
METHODS OF USE: TOPICALLY	101
METHODS OF USE: ORALLY	107
CARRIER OILS	117
RECIPES	129
OTHER BOOKS BY REBECCA PARK TOTILO	139

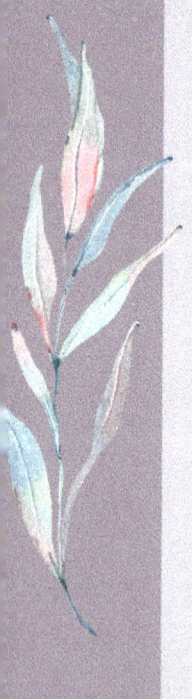

INTRODUCTION TO EMOTIONAL HEALING

Scientists have dedicated decades to studying human emotions because of their enigmatic nature and significant role in our lives. The majority of scientists concede that emotions are intricate, multi-factorial responses that can be caused by various mechanisms and stimuli. The emotions we experience are complex and mysterious because they are multi-factorial, which means they depend on multiple factors. Emotions are also complicated because any number of means or stimuli can trigger them. Simply put, emotions are your reactions to the environment surrounding you. This "environment" can comprise your physical location, the people around you, any activities you might be engaging in, and dozens of other controllable and uncontrollable factors. Your brain will analyze these factors and decide how to react emotionally. This reaction will most often result in some form of action and is generally founded on your past experiences and natural survival instincts.

People will have different emotional responses because of our unique personalities and life experiences. Individuals' personalities and experiences will influence how they perceive stimuli and their environment. This is why we each have unique responses and ways of dealing with emotions—two people can perceive the same stimuli differently.

While there are a plethora of emotions and an infinite number of reactions, emotions can generally be classified into one of two categories: positive or negative. Positive emotions can help improve your well-being and quality of life, as opposed to negative emotions, which can negatively impact your mental and physical health if they are not dealt with efficiently.

Emotions, by scientific definition, are complex responses triggered by multiple factors and stimuli. Multi-factorial responses are those that depend on several factors or causes. Mechanisms are devices, means, or methods. Stimuli are things that stimulate or incentivize a response.

POSITIVE AND NEGATIVE EMOTIONS

Any emotion we experience during the day can be classified as positive or negative. Positive emotions usually motivate us to behave in a way that will maintain that positive mood. At the same time, negative emotions can also encourage us to act in a way that will improve our mood. However, if negative emotions are left unchecked, they can have a significant impact on our health, both physical and emotional. As discussed, negative emotions can negatively affect our quality of life and even change how our body feels and functions.

HANDLING NEGATIVE EMOTIONS

It is crucial to have healthy coping mechanisms to prevent negative emotions from lowering the quality of your life. Methods of managing emotions will differ based on your personality, preferences, and other factors, as emotions vary from person to person. Some people, for example, find that physical activity or exercise helps them deal with negative emotions, while others prefer quiet reflection or meditation.

When managing negative emotions, finding a method that suits you is essential. Some options include spending time on a hobby or pastime, talking to a trusted friend or loved one, meditating, or setting aside quiet time to relax. Participating in an activity that you find enjoyable and that will help you work through negative emotions is a vital part of coping with emotions.

AROMATHERAPY THAT PROMOTES WELL-BEING

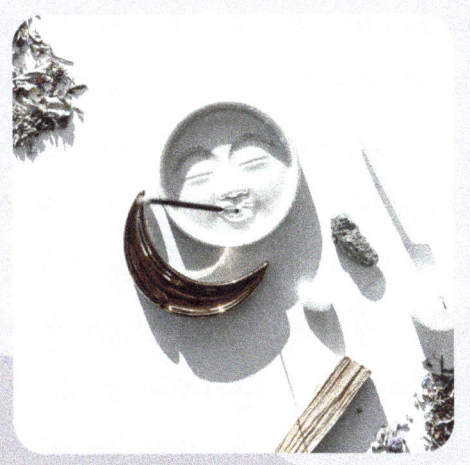

To manage moods effectively, you might want to develop healthy habits for dealing with negative emotions and incorporate essential oils into your routine. Although the coping mechanisms for negative emotions will differ from person to person, a broad selection of essential oils can be used to improve mood and promote positive feelings.

Essential oils are beneficial for emotional, spiritual, and mental healing. Aromatherapy, particularly in the use of essential oil blends, can be helpful in promoting positive emotional states of well-being and can assist in dealing with issues such as grief, anger, or frustration.

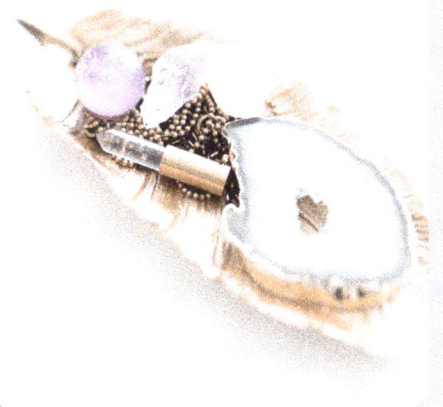

Given that each person is unique, it is beneficial to have a diverse range of oils available, each with its own individual chemical makeup, to aid in soothing, calming, or lifting one's mood. After learning how to use essential oils to improve your mood, you may find that they become a regular part of your daily routine for managing negative emotions.

> METHODS OF MANAGING EMOTIONS WILL DIFFER BASED ON YOUR PERSONALITY, PREFERENCES, AND OTHER FACTORS, AS EMOTIONS VARY FROM PERSON TO PERSON.

CHAPTER 1

USING ESSENTIAL OILS TO SUPPORT YOUR EMOTIONAL HEALTH

Essential oils have long been used for their ability to affect emotions, and they are just as helpful today for managing mood and promoting positive feelings. Those unfamiliar with the rich history of essential oils and aromatherapy might assume that using essential oils for emotions (and other purposes) is a new trend that will soon fade away. Despite this, the popularity of aromatherapy has not waned since ancient times, as essential oils have constantly proven to be an effective way of managing emotions. In addition to historical examples of aromatherapy, more recent research and scientific findings have also helped confirm essential oils' efficacy in managing mood.

The practice of using essential oils for emotional well-being, although not always called aromatherapy, dates back to ancient civilizations. People in these cultures often used plants and other plant-based materials for cooking, bathing, promoting healthy skin, and various medical treatments. In addition to these practical daily uses, essential oils were used during burials, rituals, and religious ceremonies. Ancient cultures were aware of the power plant extracts and resins had over emotions, which is why they were used so often.

Aromatherapy was widely used in ancient Greece, Rome, China, and India, often during significant events such as religious ceremonies and other rituals. For example, the Babylonians and Assyrians would burn Frankincense during religious ceremonies for its comforting smell, creating a sense of peace and relaxation. In ancient Rome, soldiers would use Fennel before battle to give them courage.

While the concept of aromatherapy has progressed and changed since ancient civilizations, it is apparent that the people

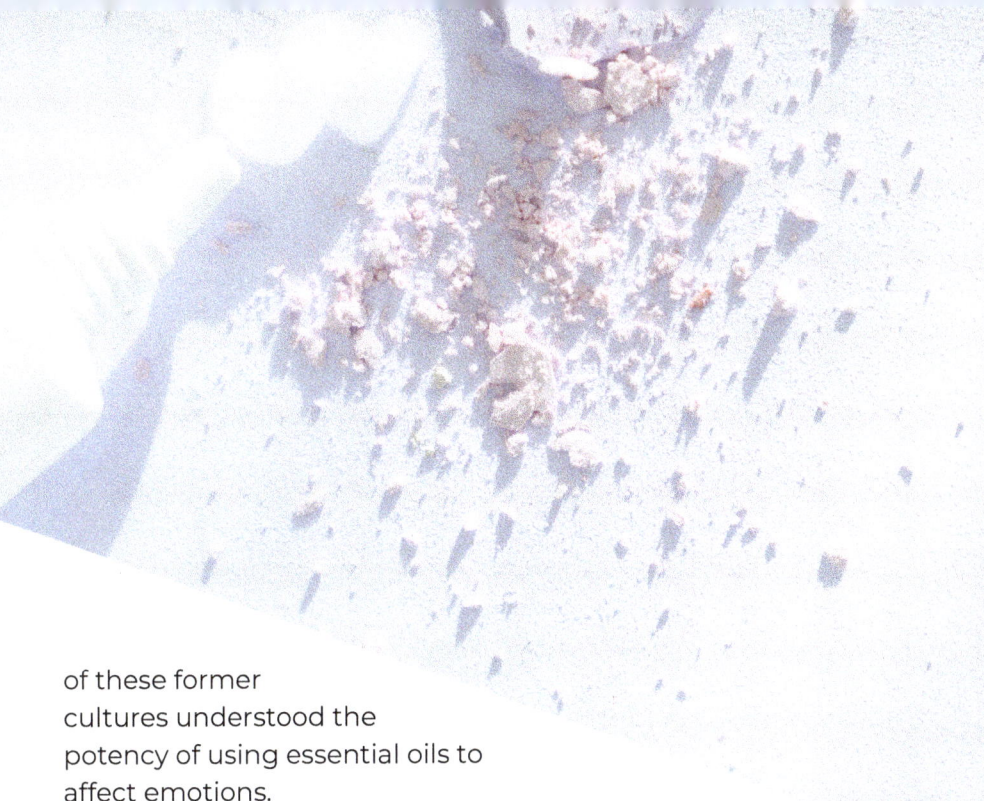

of these former cultures understood the potency of using essential oils to affect emotions.

While the practice of aromatherapy dates back centuries, it wasn't until the 20th century that the term "aromatherapy" was coined, and scientists began to support the idea of using essential oils for emotional benefit. Many people have enjoyed the benefits of aromatherapy for years, but it wasn't until the 1990s that scientists proved the connection between essential oils and mood management.

In the early 1990s, substantial research helped biologists better understand how the brain reacts to aromas. This research proved what people of ancient civilizations had already put into practice—essential oils can be used to create responses within the body, particularly to benefit and influence emotions. Although the science of emotions is largely unknown, we know there is a connection between scent and emotions. Because of this connection, aromatherapy can be a valuable tool for managing emotions and uplifting moods.

CAN AN ODOR CHANGE A PERSON'S EMOTIONS?

Can an odor really change a person's mood or emotion? According to the Bible, even God was influenced by the sense of smell. The Bible tells us that God was moved and felt compassion through the sense of smell, as in the account of Noah's offering after the flood: It says in Genesis 8:20-21,

"Then Noah built an altar to God... and offered burnt offerings... and the Lord smelled a soothing aroma and said in his heart, 'I will never again curse the ground for man's sake.'"

There may be another connection. The Hebrew word for "smell" is Reyach and shares the same root word for "spirit": Ruach. Could it be because there is life in the scent?

Even in Biblical times, essential oils were inhaled, applied to the body as anointing oil, and taken internally. The benefits extended to every aspect of their being physically, spiritually, emotionally, and mentally. The Holy Scriptures record over 1,035 references to aromatics, ointments, savors, fragrances, plants, and incense—most implying essential oils. People of the Holy Land understood the use of essential oils in maintaining wellness and physical healing, as well as the oils' ability to enhance their spiritual state in worship, prayer, and confession and for cleansing and purification from sin.

David alluded to this in Psalm 51:7 when he wrote, "Purge me with hyssop, and I will be clean: Wash me, and I will be whiter than snow." King David prayed this prayer after Nathan, the prophet, came to confront him about his sin of going into Bathsheba, committing adultery and murder (2 Samuel 12:1-4).

As he began meditating on the Law, David felt great remorse and truly repented for his sin. To restore his relationship with God, David applied his understanding of the healing properties of Hyssop as a purifier and wrote his psalm of prayer to God. Today, Hyssop is considered spiritually purifying and serves as an aid in cleansing oneself from sin, immortality, evil thoughts, or bad habits. Hyssop is also believed to repel evil spirits (angel of death), as in the case of the first Passover, when Moses asked the elders of Israel to sacrifice a spotless lamb and apply the blood to the doorposts using the branch of hyssop.

The method of using Hyssop essential oil (inhaled or applied to the skin) to purge oneself from iniquity has a scientific basis. According to David Stewart, Ph.D., D.N.M., author of "The Chemistry of Essential Oils Made Simple: God's Love Manifest in Molecules," writes that Hyssop has constituents that can reprogram the DNA where sinful tendencies (negative emotions) are stored, thus releasing and cleansing the root cause of the action.

There seems to be a connection between each essential oil's significance and its healing properties not only on an emotional level, but to every sinew of the body, corresponding with the Torah (laws or commandments in the Bible).

> THE PRACTICE OF USING ESSENTIAL OILS FOR EMOTIONAL WELL-BEING, ALTHOUGH NOT ALWAYS CALLED AROMATHERAPY, DATES BACK TO ANCIENT CIVILIZATIONS.

CHAPTER 2

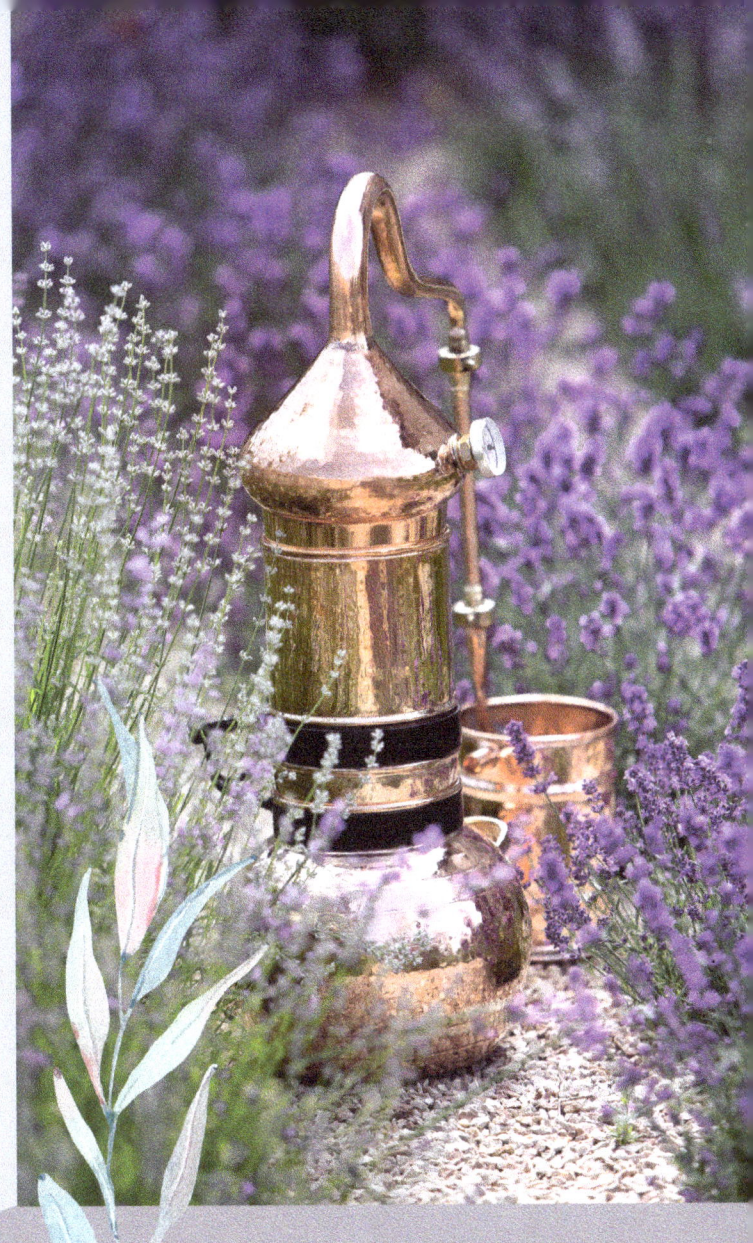

EMOTIONAL HEALING WITH OILS

There are many methods you can use to assist with your emotional healing process. You might want to pray or take some time for meditation. Here are a few suggestions for you to try, or you can come up with ones you feel would be beneficial.

Meditation: Frankincense deepens breathing. Many find this fragrance helps them enter the Creator's presence with a sense of peace. Sandalwood is another favorite used, which can be quite grounding. Diffuse either of these oils or place several drops on a candle burner on your altar.

Enhancing Discernment/Word of Knowledge: Helichrysum activates the right side of the brain, deepening intuition, while Clary Sage enhances the dreamier part of us, opening us up to receive and hear from the Creator.

Purification/Cleansing: Hyssop, Juniper, and Sage are some of the oils often used for this purpose. Many like to use these oils when moving into a new home or an existing one that they feel needs clearing out of the old. Lemon is another oil that helps bring a fresh, clean feel. You may want to diffuse or use a spray throughout the house. Make sure to open windows to clear the air. For personal use, you may want to use a few drops in your palm neat and anoint your right ear, right toe, and right thumb. Some like to add to bath water—use eight drops mixed in a tablespoon of carrier oil (vegetable) and add to running water. Soak away your worries. Add four ounces of Himalayan salts for detoxing and soak for 45 minutes.

Wounded Heart: Rose essential oil is a powerful yet gentle fragrance, allowing the hardness of past hurts and wounds to melt away. Use during times of confession. It is beneficial in cases where the heart is closed due to sadness or grief.

Releasing and Letting Go: No need to hang on to things that remind you of failure and regret. Diffuse Frankincense and inhale deeply. With each exhale, allow each negative thought to leave you.

Final Hour and Bereavement: In the case of someone's passing into the afterlife, several essential oils are used. Melissa is the oil traditionally associated with easing this final transition. You may want to diffuse in a candle or burner to offer them support and comfort. Spikenard may be used on the body in preparing the person for their final resting place. For family and friends, other oils such as Rose, Neroli, and Lavender may be used for grief and shock, and Cypress for times of loss and needed strength.

Spiritual Protection: Rosemary, Hyssop, Juniper, and Fennel are all oils that have a history of use in times of spiritual warfare. In medieval times, Fennel was used to ward off evil spirits, while Juniper cleanses and protects. Rosemary supports insulating yourself from unwanted influences that might arise during your day. Place several drops in the palm of your hand and rub them on your body, stroking downwards. An aromatherapist instructor suggested making a blend of these oils to apply to the solar plexus area since that is often where negative energy enters the body.

Entering In and Worship: All Biblical fragrances, such as Frankincense, Sandalwood, Cypress, Cedarwood, etc., enhance your time with God. These help to quiet the mind and bring things into focus. Using fragrances reserved only for this time helps to set the tone and make it a "set apart" time for you and the Creator alone.

"

NO NEED TO HANG ON TO THINGS THAT REMIND YOU OF FAILURE AND REGRET. DIFFUSE FRANKINCENSE AND INHALE DEEPLY. WITH EACH EXHALE, ALLOW EACH NEGATIVE THOUGHT TO LEAVE YOU.

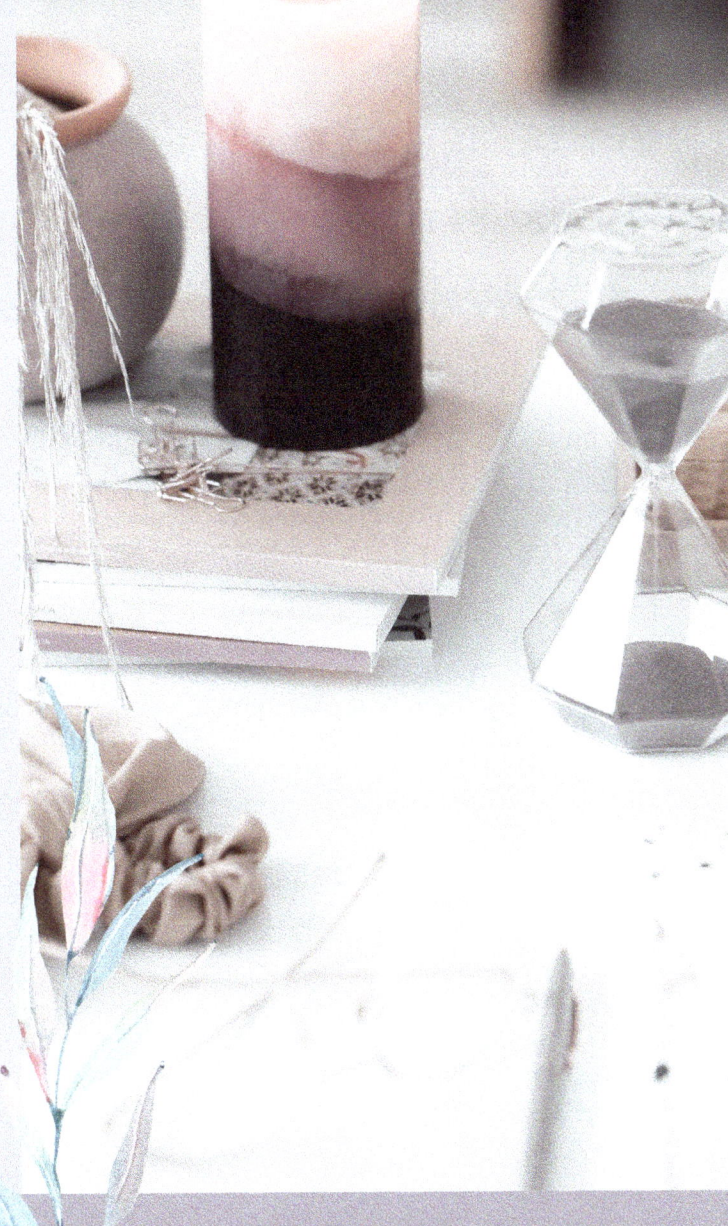

CHAPTER 3

WHY USE ESSENTIAL OILS FOR MOODS

Although the science of emotions is still largely mysterious, we know there is a connection between scent and emotions. As mentioned, each person experiences feelings differently; therefore, the method used for managing emotions will vary from person to person. Many options are available for coping with negative emotions; you will discover several benefits of using essential oils to manage emotions.

Depending on the individual and the emotion, various methods exist for changing or managing a mood. However, several of these choices are not beneficial for your physical health. Regrettably, some people utilize dicey or even perilous methods to change or manage their emotions, which can result in more troublesome issues later on.

The advantage of using essential oils to maintain one's mood is that they relieve, tranquilize, and raise emotions naturally. Pure, high-grade essential oils are powerful, so only a tiny amount is needed to produce the desired outcome. Essential oils are powerful yet safe to use as they come from natural sources. Aromatherapy is an excellent alternative to many of the other mood management programs out there.

As we discussed, high-quality essential oils are potent. Usually, you will start to feel some response as soon as you open the bottle and smell the oil. This power and potency mean that you will only need to use a small amount of oil to help manage your mood.

Essential oils create natural, favorable responses, making them more reliable for managing emotions than other methods. With aromatherapy, you can harness the power of essential oils to help you manage the range of emotions you feel every day.

People experience emotions differently, so the methods for managing emotions will vary from person to person. There are many options available for improving one's mood and coping with negative emotions, and what's more, there are several benefits to using aromatherapy and essential oils to manage emotions.

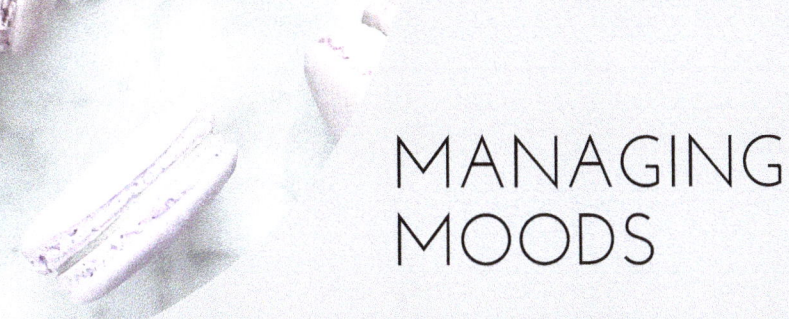

MANAGING MOODS

Aromatherapy has remained a popular method of managing mood throughout history for several reasons, one of which is its simplicity. Once you learn about essential oils and how they work, you can easily incorporate them into your daily routine to help improve your mood. After reading the proper methods for applying essential oils and understanding which oils possess relaxing, calming, uplifting, invigorating, or other properties, it will be effortless to enjoy the emotional benefits of aromatherapy.

Due to their easy application, essential oils can be used alongside other mood management techniques to help you maintain control of your emotions. Essential oils are frequently used with practices like massage or meditation and can even be used in activities such as exercise, bathing, or sleeping. Customizing essential oils and aromatherapy to your preferences can ease negative emotions during your daily routine.

Essential oils are not only beneficial for physical healing but are emotionally, spiritually, and mentally healing as well. Aromatherapy, particularly in essential oil blends, can be extremely useful in promoting positive emotional states of well-being and can assist in dealing with issues such as grief, anger, or frustration.

People who experience stress daily may find using essential oil blends helpful for calming their nerves and

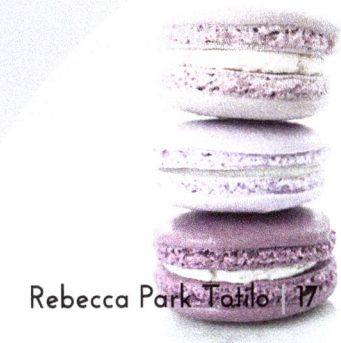

help in promoting a less stressful environment. One of the reasons why aromatherapy works so well in this particular situation is that essential oils' molecules are easily inhaled, which allows them to be fast-acting and quickly absorbed into the body. The molecules released through aromatherapy stimulate and affect portions of the brain that can trigger specific types of emotions in the brain or soothe other less desirable types of emotions. Stress compromises normal body function due to physiological and psychological factors. It is multidimensional and can affect the body, soul, and spirit. The impact psychologically can manifest as depression, undue worry, and psychosis, among others. Physiological impact results in the body being unable to respond to demands made on it effectively, which ultimately results in impaired metabolism and defective tissue repair processes. This usually occurs when the coping mechanisms are overwhelmed. A healthy person with good social support is able to cope with the stress better, and the contrast suffers more in comparison. When the body undergoes long-term stress, its coping mechanisms become progressively less competent. Stress also increases the body's energy demand due to hormonal imbalance and increased metabolic rate.

Essential oils can be used to modulate the stress response and bring a calming effect to the body. Cypress, Cedarwood, Chamomile, Coriander, Ginger, and Frankincense, among others, have this effect.

Of course, not all essential oils will affect everyone in the same manner. Other memories associated with particular types of aromas may affect how the aroma will impact their emotional state of being. For instance, if you have a particularly strong emotional response to a specific type of oil or scent, this will affect its ability to positively influence your emotional well-being. If Cinnamon, usually a warm and comforting scent, has become associated with the death of a family member, you are less likely to be positively influenced by Cinnamon essential oil.

CHAPTER 4

THE SCIENTIFIC EVIDENCE BEHIND AROMATHERAPY

Aromatherapy has been a successful method of impacting emotions for centuries, and the connection between the brain and scent is more than an ancient belief. There is now scientific evidence to support it. This is the result of extensive research and many discoveries. The science behind what makes aromatherapy work explains how different aromas can elicit certain feelings. In this chapter, we will look at the scientific basis for aromatherapy to better understand how essential oils affect emotions and influence mood.

HOW THE BRAIN PROCESSES AROMAS

Whenever we inhale a distinct aroma (like the scent of an essential oil), it will be processed by different parts of the brain in a specific sequence. The olfactory membranes, with almost 800 million nerve endings, receive the micro-fine, vaporized oil particles and carry them along the axon of the nerve fibers, connecting them with the secondary neurons in the olfactory bulb. The impulses are then transported to the limbic system and the olfactory sensory center at the base of the brain. They then pass between the pituitary and pineal glands and move to the amygdala—the memory center. The impulses travel to the gustatory center, where the sensation of taste is perceived.

The olfactory system is linked to the limbic system, where our emotions and memories are kept. Because of this connection to the limbic system, we respond to a scent based on any memories we have associated with that smell. The response generated by the limbic system often causes an immediate flood of emotions, otherwise known as an emotional response. Given that our sense of smell is closely linked to the area of the brain that encodes memories and emotions, it is understandable why particular smells evoke specific emotions. The benefit of using aromatherapy for emotional help is that you get to select which essential oils you want to trigger desired emotions, especially when attempting to improve or eliminate negative emotions.

The part of the nose responsible for odor detection, called the olfactory, sends impulses created by various odors to the amygdala, which also serves as the memory center of our brain for fear and trauma. The discovery how significant role the amygdala plays in storing and releasing emotional trauma wasn't discovered until 1989, and ONLY odor or fragrance stimulation has a profound effect in triggering a response with this gland.

Comprehending the delicate chemistry of each essential oil allows us to control our emotions and manage our moods by producing a precise reaction in the brain.

THE LIMBIC SYSTEM

The limbic system—often referred to as the "emotional brain"—is located in the cerebrum. This part of the brain is in charge of emotional responses, hormone function, behavior, motivation, long-term memory, and sense of smell. There are several other specialized areas in the limbic system, such as:

- Hippocampus: responsible for forming short- and long-term memories.
- Amygdala: perceives emotions such as anger, fear, and sadness; plays a role in controlling aggression; helps store memories of events and emotions; also plays a role in sexual activity and libido.
- Hypothalamus: controls reproduction, sleep patterns, and body homeostasis.
- Thalamus: relays sensory information to the cerebral cortex.

Not only are our emotions closely related to our sense of smell, but this also explains why our emotions can profoundly impact other areas of our lives. The part of the brain that controls emotions is also involved in memory, sexual desire, reproduction, sleep, and maintaining equilibrium.

The exact details of how smells affect emotions are challenging to pinpoint. But if we think about what happens when we inhale an aroma, we can begin to understand the connection.

When an odorant molecule enters your nose, it lands on tiny hairs called cilia. The cilia then start to vibrate, creating an electrical signal. The signal travels to a receptor cell, which starts to bundle packets of smell information. The smell information is then further bundled into packets that travel to the limbic system via pyramidal cells.

The limbic system is responsible for emotional responses to smells. For example, we all know the experience of smelling something that triggers a memory, such as your grandmother's perfume.

Although the emotional response mechanism is not entirely clear, it is evident that it exists. Research shows that olfactory-evoked memories often create a more significant emotional arousal than simply recalling a memory with no associated olfactory stimuli. Since emotions and olfaction have a direct relationship in the brain, essential oils can help unlock stored memories and emotions. When you breathe in an essential oil, molecules enter the limbic system and elicit an emotional response. For instance, personal feelings towards a particular oil may go beyond preferring one scent over another. It could be that the oil is triggering an emotional response. Essential oils that create positive emotions are more likely to be favored because aromas actually affect brain waves and emotions.

PLANT SOURCE

The chemical makeup of an essential oil is determined by many factors, with the plant source being one of the most important. The type of plant the oil comes from will largely determine the chemical constituents present in the oil. This, in turn, will affect the benefits the oil can provide. To learn more about how plant source and chemical profile can determine the benefits of an essential oil, please see the plant categories below.

Mint: Mint essential oils typically contain a high concentration of ketones and are considered energizing, invigorating, and uplifting.

Floral: Floral essential oils are composed chiefly of monoterpene alcohols and esters and promote calming and toning benefits.

Citrus: Citrus oils contain monoterpenes known as limonene and beta-pinene and typically have strong uplifting characteristics.

Tree, Grass, Herb: Essential oils from trees, herbs, and grasses are rich in esters, oxides, and sesquiterpenes. These oils are generally soothing, renewing, and grounding.

Spice: Essential oils from spices are beneficial for their warming properties and consist of phenol chemical constituents.

ESSENTIAL OIL CHEMICAL CONSTITUENTS SUMMARY

Aldehydes – antifungal, anti-inflammatory, antiviral, **calming**, **sedative** (Lemongrass, Citronella, Melissa, Eucalyptus)

Esters – antifungal, anti-inflammatory, antispasmodic, equilibrating, **sedative**, and **calming for the nervous system** (Roman Chamomile, Clary Sage, Lavender)

Ethers – antispasmodic, balancing, carminative (Tarragon, Aniseed, Basil)

Ketones – antiviral, analgesic, cell-regenerating, cooling, decongestant, promote tissue formation, powerful mucolytic, **stimulating or calming depending on the amount used**, neurotoxic (Eucalyptus, Helichrysum, Hyssop, Rosemary, Sage)

Lactones – **balancing**, decongestant, photosensitive (Bergamot)

Monoterpene Alcohols – anti-infectious, antiseptic, antiviral, bactericidal, diuretic, immune stimulant (Lavender, Marjoram, Peppermint, Petitgrain, Rosewood, Tea Tree)

Monoterpene Hydrocarbons – antiseptic, antiviral, decongestant, rubefacient, possible skin irritant (Juniper Berry, Pine, and most citrus oils)

Oxides – antiviral, decongestant, diuretic, expectorant, immune stimulant, **mentally stimulating**, powerful healer for the respiratory system (Eucalyptus and most oils in the Myrtaceae family)

Phenols – analgesic, anti-infectious, anti-inflammatory, antiviral, **stimulating**, strong antibacterial, hot oils, immune-stimulating (Oregano, Thyme, Winter Savory)

Sesquiterpene Alcohols – anti-allergenic, anti-inflammatory, cooling, **grounding**, immune stimulant (German Chamomile, Sandalwood, Rose)

Sesquiterpene Hydrocarbons – anti-allergenic, anti-inflammatory, antispasmodic, cicatrisant, cooling, **sedative** (German Chamomile, Helichrysum, Yarrow)

CHEMICAL CONSTITUENTS EMOTIONAL EFFECT CHART

Calming	Aldehydes, Coumarins, Ethers, Esters, Sesquiterpenes
Energizing	Alcohols
Toning	Alcohols
Sedative	Aldehydes, Coumarins, Ethers
Stimulating	Alcohols, Ethers, Ketones, Monoterpenes, Monoterpenols, Oxides, Phenols, Terpenes
Balancing	Ethers, Esters, Alcohols
Cooling	Aldehydes, Esters
Hypnotic	Esters, Lactones
Relaxing	Aldehydes, Coumarins, Ethers, Esters, Lactones, Sesquiterpenes
Soothing	Aldehydes, Ethers, Esters
Warming	Phenols, Oxides, Terpenes

WHEN YOU LACK MOTIVATION, ENTHUSIASM, OR INSPIRATION, CHOOSE AN ESSENTIAL OIL WITH AN UPLIFTING CHEMICAL PROFILE TO HELP YOU OUT OF A FUNK. WHEN YOU FEEL FRAZZLED, OVERWHELMED, OR DOWN, USE A CALMING OIL TO HELP PROMOTE SOOTHING, GROUNDING, OR RENEWED EMOTIONS.

STIMULATING AND SOOTHING OILS

Scientific research has revealed that certain chemical constituents in essential oils make some oils stimulating and others soothing that have a calming effect on the nervous system. Every essential oil has a different chemical composition, but they can all be categorized as uplifting or calming based on their chemical constituents. This is what makes essential oils so beneficial for managing emotions.

Recent studies by Pierre Franchomme and Daniel Penoel have found that essential oils possess positive and negative charges ascribed to the main chemical groups. For instance, Phenylpropanes, commonly known as warming and potent stimulants, have been attributed with a positive charge. At the same time, Aldehydes that are considered cooling with calming sedative effects on the central nervous system (including both the sympathetic and parasympathetic systems) possess a negative charge. Simply put, these chemicals affect receptors in the body by stimulating or soothing.

Stimulating	Soothing
Acids	Alcohols
Alcohols	Aldehydes
Phenols	Coumarins
Phenylpropanes	Ethers
Terpenes	Esters
Hydrocarbons	

STIMULATING ESSENTIAL OILS

Stimulating oils are best described as uplifting, refreshing, perky, lively, energizing, invigorating, and warming. Some oils may go either way, with the ability to be stimulating or soothing, depending on the other oils in that blend. Uplifting essential oils, mostly made of ketones, phenols, and monoterpenes like beta-pinene and limonene, can raise your spirits, promote energy, or make you feel warmer. Below is a list of uplifting essential oils.

Top	Middle	Base
Ajowan	Balsam Fir	Angelica Root
Anise Star	Bay	Ginger
Aniseed	Black Pepper	Jasmine
Basil	Blue Tansy	Myrrh
Camphor	Cardamom	Nutmeg
Cedar Leaf	Caraway Seed	Patchouli
Celery	Carrot Seed	Tarragon
Citronella	Cinnamon	
Coriander	Clove Bud	
Eucalyptus	Dill	
Fennel	Elemi	
Galbanum	Fir	
Grapefruit	Geranium	
Lemon	Hyssop	
Lime	Juniper Berry	
Mandarin	Lavender	
Orange	Marjoram	
Oregano	Myrtle	

Palmarosa	Niaouli
Peppermint	Nutmeg
Lemon Verbena	Pine
Sage	Pimento Leaf
Spearmint	Rosemary
Tea Tree	Thyme
Rosemary Verbena	

SOOTHING ESSENTIAL OILS

Soothing oils are best described as sedative, grounding, balancing, relaxing and supportive. Essential oils that have a calming effect typically contain monoterpene alcohols, sesquiterpenes, esters, and oxides. Below is a list of calming oils that promote soothing, grounding, or rejuvenating emotions.

Top	Middle	Base
Bergamot	Balsam Fir	Balsam
Cajeput	Cardamom	Benzoin
Citronella	Chamomile, Roman	Cedarwood
Clary Sage	Cypress	Cistus Labdanum
Coriander	Fir Needle	Frankincense
Grapefruit	Geranium	Ginger
Lemongrass	Hyssop	Jasmine
Niaouli	Lavender	Myrrh
Orange	Linden Blossom	Opoponax
Petitgrain	Marjoram	Patchouli
Spearmint	Melissa	Rose
Tangerine	Myrtle	Rosewood
Tea Tree	Neroli	Sandalwood
	Nutmeg	Spikenard
	Palmarosa	Tarragon
	Thyme	Valerian
		Vanilla
		Vetiver
		Violet
		Ylang Ylang

Rebecca Park Totilo

> UPLIFTING ESSENTIAL OILS, MOSTLY MADE OF KETONES, PHENOLS, AND MONOTERPENES LIKE BETA-PINENE AND LIMONENE, CAN RAISE YOUR SPIRITS, PROMOTE ENERGY, OR MAKE YOU FEEL WARMER.

CHAPTER 5 —

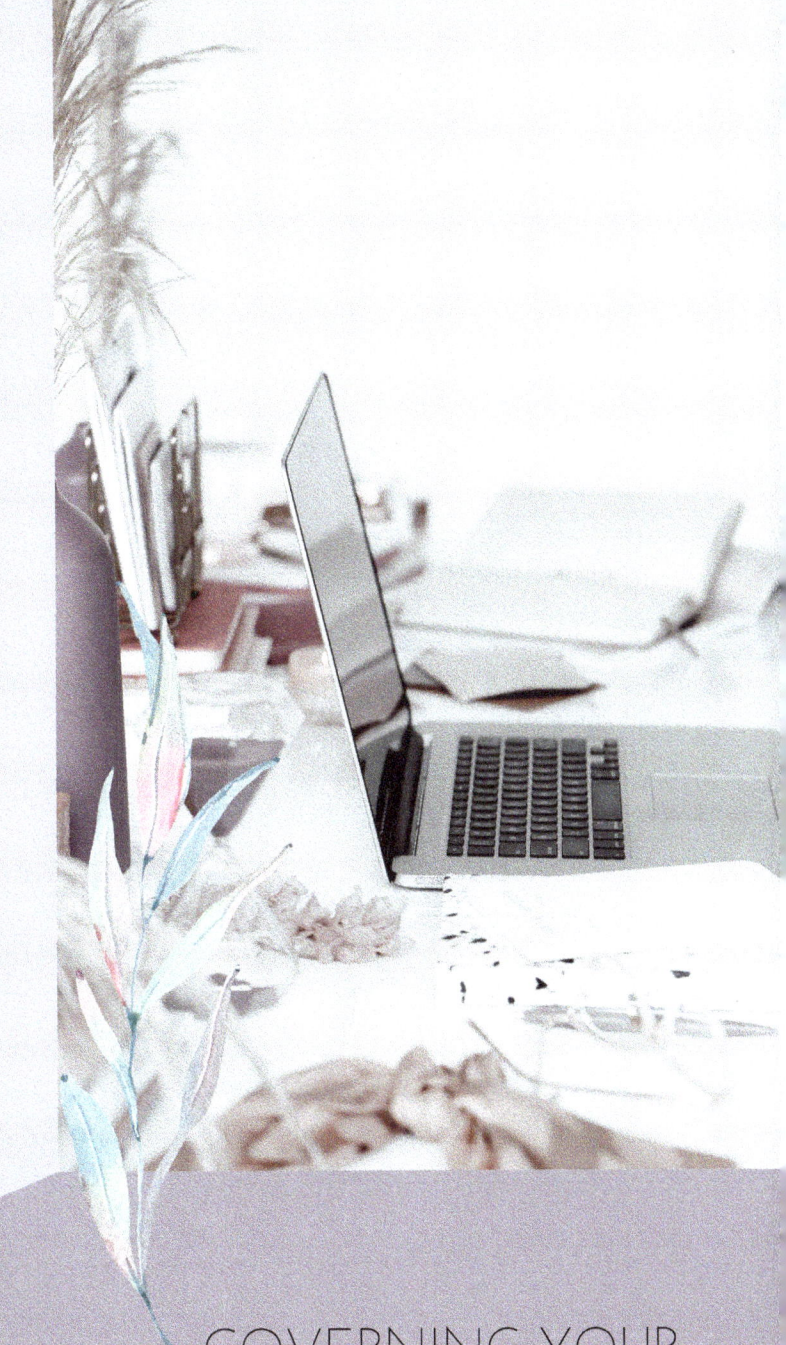

GOVERNING YOUR EMOTIONAL RESPONSE

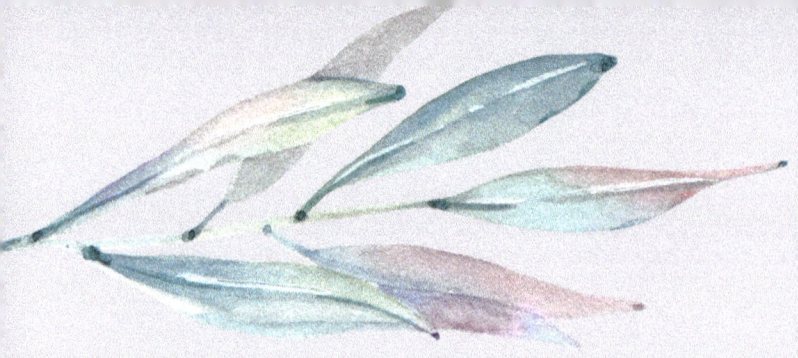

Aromatherapy lets individuals utilize particular oils to induce specific emotional responses and govern their moods. However, as no two individuals are completely alike, neither are people's reactions to smells. This is because aromas are processed in the limbic system, where our memories and emotions are kept. Therefore, two people can experience different feelings toward the smell of the same oil. While an essential oil can generate a particular response, we must remember that our reaction to an aroma is based on our experiences, preferences, environment, and even our genes.

TRIGGERING MEMORIES

A scent can elicit specific emotions by triggering memories that can cause emotional responses. Even though everyone has different memories and backgrounds, we can still use the power of essential oils to create the desired response. Each essential oil has a different chemical makeup, which gives the oil its unique properties and benefits. The chemical makeup of the essential oil will determine its attributes, benefits, and what kind of emotional responses it can produce. Therefore, it is possible to choose an essential oil based on its chemical profile to elicit a specific emotional response.

This is part of the reason why aromatherapy has been around for so long—individuals can create a bespoke aromatic experience based on their own unique experiences and preferences. No two people will have the same reaction to a single oil, which makes aromatherapy a very personalized way of dealing with emotions. Your personal experiences, feelings, and preferences will dictate how an essential oil helps you, making it easy to customize your aromatherapy experience to your particular needs.

THE EMOTIONAL EXPERIENCE

Emotions are complex occurrences that can be most simply understood as a combination of physical sensations and thought patterns. In this section, you will discover how to recognize your feeling and separate yourself from their power. Once this is done, you can use your oils to let go of your negative emotions rather than allowing them to rule you.

- Take a few moments to become aware of your body and the feelings you are experiencing.
- Try to recall as many details as possible about the recent event that triggered this emotion.
- Close your eyes to visualize the experience. Identify the feeling in your body.

UNDERSTANDING YOUR EMOTIONS

When you are experiencing this emotion, investigate it closely. What feeling best describes what you are feeling? Check the list of emotions in this book to identify the one you are experiencing if unsure.

Pay attention to where you feel it in the body. Where you experience the feeling or sensation in your body helps you to know which method of use for your essential oil blend is best for this feeling. For instance, a massage blend may be the best delivery method if you feel stress in the shoulders or back.

Tune in to the mental state that accompanies this physical sensation. As you recognize the feeling, what is happening in the mind? It may be a time when you were stressed, anxious, frustrated, or sad. Try not to "relive the event" but investigate the feeling.

Feelings are closely related to thoughts. You will want to explore this further once the specific event does not easily trigger you, especially if you have a tendency to "relive" feelings due to your mind replaying the event repeatedly.

Investigate this experience in both mind and body, resting with each for a few minutes. Now, gather your oils for the specific feeling and choose one or two oils to use. Open each one and take a deep breath.

Allow the mind to relax for a few deep breaths before opening the eyes.

You may want to prepare blends for specific emotions you experience regularly.

WHAT TO DO WITH NEGATIVE EMOTIONS

The following tips can help you when experiencing negative emotions.

- Keep your mind and emotions under control. The Bible reminds us to cast down evil imaginations and bring every thought under control. In other words, you can't let every thought that strays into your mind dictate your feelings. Don't even entertain thoughts that you know will upset you.
- Dwell only on sweet, loving thoughts of Hope. Ruminate only on things that are pure and of good report. It is okay to recall an event that upset you, but you will want to deal with it immediately so that it doesn't take a foothold in your heart and cause mental torture.
- Practice gratitude every moment. Remember to be

thankful for everything—even when it's not necessarily the answer you were looking for. Even in difficult situations, there is a lesson to be learned.
- Do not dwell on negative emotions such as grief or anger. Feelings like these should not be suppressed either, though. Acknowledge them, then release them.

To achieve this, create a simple ritual for releasing negative emotions until there is no more negativity to give away. After releasing each negative emotion, replace those feelings with love, joy, and gratitude, acknowledging the act by inhaling an essential oil you love. Continue to use the oils and inhale them frequently as a cleansing, transformative reminder to support your positive emotional outlook. You may want to use different oils when dealing with multiple emotional issues. You may select them purely on intuition or refer to the list of emotions here for a particular issue.

SEASONAL DEPRESSION DISORDER

Various essential oils possess properties that help deal with a range of emotional states. For example, some of the best essential oils for helping with the winter blues and depression are scents of citrus oils to help warm the spirit. Here are some examples:

Bergamot essential oil is a great choice when dealing with depression and anxiety and is the first choice for Seasonal Affective Disorder. It's simple and heart-warming, and the pleasant fragrance is excellent for dreary, long winter days.

Sweet Orange is suitable for brightening your day and is gentle enough for children. It is excellent for anxiety, stress, and insomnia.

Lemon helps to prevent emotional outbursts and aids in making decisions, helping to bring mental clarity.

> VARIOUS ESSENTIAL OILS POSSESS PROPERTIES THAT HELP DEAL WITH A RANGE OF EMOTIONAL STATES.

CHAPTER 6

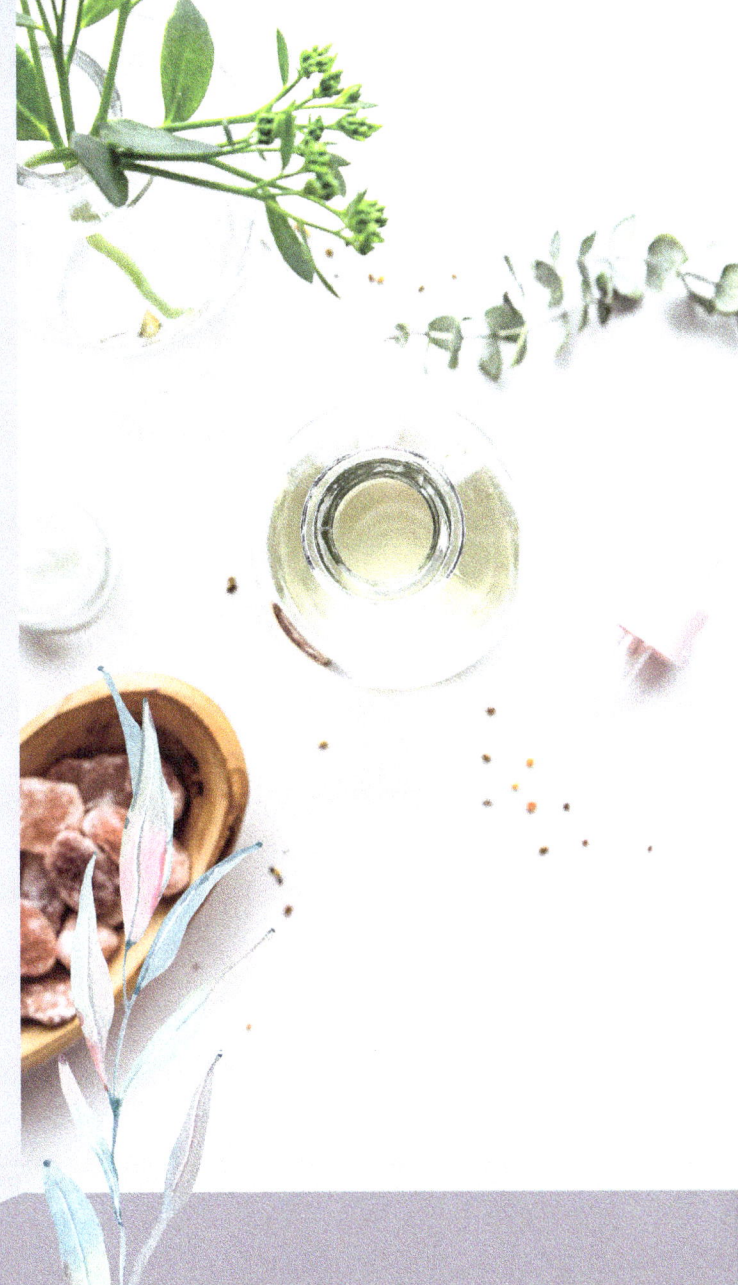

ESSENTIAL OILS FOR EMOTIONS

Now that you better understand the scientific principles that make essential oils effective for influencing emotions, let's look at how to use essential oils to manage your mood. Understanding each oil's benefits is key to experiencing successful mood management using essential oils. Each essential oil's unique chemical profile determines its characteristics and benefits. As you study each oil, its chemical structure, and its benefits for emotions, you can choose the right oil (or a combination of multiple oils) to create the desired emotional response.

When creating blending for emotional issues, you will want to choose essential oils with pleasant scents. Emotional issues can be effectively treated with diffusion, but other methods, such as a gentle massage or warm bath, may also be beneficial.

If you are already familiar with essential oils, you probably know of several oils that promote relaxation or are energizing. For instance, studies have shown that Valerian essential oil is more effective in relaxation than prescribed medication. Adding a few drops of a relaxing essential oil to a diffuser is one of the easiest ways to experience healing.

Of course, essential oils are not one size fits all. What may work for some people may not work for others. This is because essential oils are adaptogens and affect people differently. Be flexible and try other essential oils until you find which oils work best.

Basil

Basil *(Ocimum basilicum)* is used to relieve mental fatigue, anxiety, and depression. It is incredibly soothing and uplifting and is popular with massage therapists for alleviating tension and stress in their patients. Basil is an excellent insect repellent when diluted, with linalool's mild analgesic properties. It is also highly effective as an antispasmodic, antiemetic, and carminative. Diffuse Basil oil to lessen feelings of anxiousness. This oil may irritate sensitive skin. Avoid use during pregnancy.

Usage: Oral, Topical, Inhalation
Note: Top

Bergamot

Bergamot *(Citrus bergamia)* is a favorite oil for treating depression. Studies have shown that Bergamot oil can reduce anxiety and improve mood. It is thought to reduce the presence of cortisol in saliva, which gives it its sedative properties. The therapeutic properties of Bergamot include acting as an antidepressant and calmative. Unlike many other citrus oils that may be energizing, Bergamot is calming, reduces stress and anxiety, and possesses sedative qualities. Bergamot is known to slow the heart rate and lower blood pressure. Bergamot is calming and uplifting, making it an excellent oil for reducing feelings of negativity. Bergamot's soothing property helps the body relax and heal. Bergamot essential oil has phototoxic properties; therefore, exposure to the sun should be avoided after use.

Usage: Oral, Topical, Inhalation
Note: Top

Blue Tansy

Blue Tansy *(Tanacetum annuum)*, also called Moroccan Chamomile, has a surprisingly sweet scent making it ideal for applications in skin care products and skin therapies. Blue Tansy contains the active azulene, best known for its skin care properties and as an anti-inflammatory agent. This oil induces relaxation, reduces nervous tension and stress, and has hormone-like actions stimulating the thymus gland. It helps to stabilize blood sugar, eliminates bruises, itching, rashes, and cysts, and reduces blood pressure. Its therapeutic properties include anthelmintic, carminative, antispasmodic, stimulant, tonic, antipruritic, emmenagogue, and hypotensive. Particular attention should be given to its blue color as it may change cream or lotion colors. Blue Tansy essential oil is generally non-irritating and non-toxic. Avoid use during pregnancy.

Usage: Topical, Inhalation
Note: Middle

Camphor, White

White Camphor *(Cinnamomum camphora)* is known to be clarifying, energizing, and purifying. The chemical constituents of Camphor are carminative and laxative properties. Camphor has been used to treat nervous depression, acne, inflammation, arthritis, and muscular aches and pains. Camphor oil is a powerful oil and should be used with caution. Overdosing can cause convulsions and vomiting. Pregnant women or persons who have epilepsy and asthma should not use it.

Usage: Topical
Note: Top

Cananga

Cananga *(Cananga odorata)* is sought for its aphrodisiac, antidepressant, sedative, and tonic properties. While this oil is non-toxic, it may be sensitizing; for that reason, use well diluted.

Usage: Topical, Inhalation
Note: Middle

Cardamom

Cardamom *(Elettaria cardamomum)* is an uplifting oil. Cardamom is also helpful for muscle cramps, catarrh, and physical exhaustion. It is best used in baths, massage oils, lotions, and a diffuser. For the body, its stimulating nature warms sore muscles and supports circulation. For the mind, it improves mental clarity and uplifts one's spirit. Cardamom is known to warm the heart, with a long history of being used as an aphrodisiac. The unmistakable, refreshing aroma of Cardamom oil can help promote a positive mood. It is non-toxic, non-irritant, and non-sensitizing. Please check with your healthcare provider before use during pregnancy.

Usage: Oral, Topical, Inhalation
Note: Middle

Cedarwood

Cedarwood *(Cedrus atlantica)* contains therapeutic properties that are tonic and sedative. Like Lavender, Cedarwood is considered suitable for detoxifying and clearing negative emotions. Because inhaling Cedarwood triggers the release of serotonin in the brain, which converts to melatonin, the essential oil is known for its sedative qualities and usefulness in treating insomnia. Use Cedarwood oil aromatically to help relax the mind and body. Cedarwood has been shown to decrease heart rate and blood pressure, maintaining its effectiveness as a sleep aid and alleviating hypertension and anxiety. It is considered a non-toxic and non-irritant oil. It is a relaxing and soothing oil that allows the brain to stop processing.

Usage: Topical, Inhalation
Note: Base

Roman Chamomile

Roman Chamomile *(Chamaemelum nobile)* is another popular oil for encouraging relaxation. This oil promotes feelings of peace and calm. There are several species of Chamomile, but Roman Chamomile (Anthemis nobilis aka Chamaemelum nobile) essential oil is the most potent for battling anxiety. Roman Chamomile is an ancient herb with therapeutic properties, including sedative and relaxing. It is recommended to treat insomnia, stress, and nervous tension, so it is an excellent choice to help you relax. The therapeutic properties of Roman Chamomile oil are analgesic, antispasmodic, antidepressant, antineuralgic, antiphlogistic, carminative, emmenagogue, sedative, nervine, tonic, and vulnerary. It is non-toxic and non-irritant. Roman Chamomile's ability to act as a mild sedative to ease nerves and decrease anxiety to treat conditions like hysteria, nightmares, insomnia and other sleep difficulties has also been researched. While the root of these effects is not determined, they appear to be psychological. Studies also have shown Chamomile's effectiveness in relieving stress and anxiety. It has a warm, sweet, herbaceous scent that is relaxing and calming for both mind and body. Roman Chamomile's gentleness makes it especially useful for restless children.

Usage: Oral, Topical, Inhalation
Note: Middle

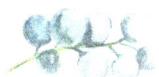

German Chamomile

German Chamomile *(Matricaria chamomilla)* is a relaxing and rejuvenating agent that calms nerves, reduces stress, and aids insomnia. German Chamomile is known for its anti-inflammatory abilities and can help alleviate muscle spasms and joint pain. Its therapeutic properties include analgesic, anti-convulsive, antidepressant, cholagogue, diuretic, emmenagogue, nervine, sedative, tonic, and vasoconstrictor. Azulene gives this oil its intense blue color, while sesquiterpenes lend its calming effect. German Chamomile calms nerves, eases headaches, and aids in relaxation. It operates as a mild tranquilizer and as a sleep inducer. German Chamomile impacts the same areas of the brain and nervous system as popular anti-anxiety medications and can also assist in minimizing aches and pains. Its calming reputation and stress-reducing effects are due to apigenin, which Chamomile contains and is known to bind to benzodiazepine receptors. Of course, the benefits of German Chamomile are not restricted to the use of its essential oil. The plant's flower can be enjoyed as a relaxing hot drink when brewed as tea.

Usage: Oral, Topical, Inhalation
Note: Middle

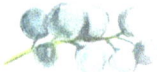

Clary Sage

Clary Sage *(Salvia sclarea)* can be used as an antidepressant and as a sedative. Women experiencing hormonal changes or menopause symptoms such as hot flashes find this oil beneficial. Clary Sage's properties are antidepressant, anticonvulsive, antispasmodic, anti-inflammatory, aphrodisiac, carminative, euphoric, hypotensive, nervine, sedative, and nerve tonic. Clary Sage oil is non-toxic and non-sensitizing. Its anti-inflammatory and antispasmodic properties help to calm and soothe the body and mind. Clary Sage is a natural sedative that may reduce your cortisol levels, known as the stress hormone. Do not use it during pregnancy or if you are at risk for breast cancer, as it may have an estrogen-like effect on the body. Clary Sage is similar to Valerian in that it affects the GABA receptors, which help reduce stress. Clary Sage is known to create a restful environment while reducing feelings of anxiousness. Clary Sage also has mood-lifting properties that are useful in treating patients who suffer from depression. When this oil was compared to others, such as Chamomile and Lavender, it was the most effective at combating stress.

Usage: Oral, Topical, Inhalation
Note: Top-Middle

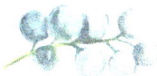

Clove Bud

Clove Bud *(Syzygium aromaticum)* has a spicy, rich scent and is used for its stimulating and energizing properties. Clove helps to prevent vomiting and other disturbances due to emotional upsets. Clove oil's therapeutic properties are analgesic, antiseptic, antispasmodic, antineuralgic, carminative, anti-infectious, disinfectant, insecticide, tonic, stomachic, uterine, and stimulant. This oil may cause sensitization in some individuals and should be used in dilution. Avoid use during pregnancy.

Usage: Oral, Topical, Inhalation
Note: Middle

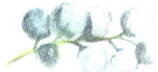

Cilantro or Coriander

Cilantro or Coriander *(Coriandrum sativum)* works as an analgesic, carminative, revitalizing, and stimulating oil. It relieves mental fatigue, migraine pain, stress, and nervous debility. Coriander's warming effect helps alleviate pain such as rheumatism, arthritis, and muscle spasms. Coriander oil can be diffused to promote feelings of calmness and relaxation. The healing properties of Cilantro or Coriander oil are attributed to phytonutrient content, including carvone, geraniol, limonene, borneol, camphor, elemol, and linalool. Coriander is traditionally used in India for its anti-inflammatory properties.

Usage: Oral, Topical, Inhalation
Note: Top

Cypress

Cypress *(Cupressus)* oil calms and soothes anger while having a positive effect on one's mood. It is suitable for various female problems and good for coughs and bronchitis. Cypress assists with bodily fluids by improving circulation. Its properties include antibacterial, anti-infectious, anti-inflammatory, anti-rheumatic, antiseptic, antispasmodic, astringent, decongestant, diuretic, and vein tonic. Avoid long-term use with high-blood pressure.

Usage: Topical, Inhalation
Note: Middle-Base

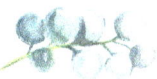

Cypress, Blue

Blue Cypress *(Callitris columellaris var intratropica)* is considered similar to German Chamomile due to its soothing and relaxing properties for the nerves without having sedative properties. The therapeutic properties of Cypress are astringent, antiseptic, antispasmodic, deodorant, diuretic, hemostatic, hepatic, styptic, sudorific, vasoconstrictor, respiratory tonic, and sedative. It is considered non-toxic and non-irritant. Blue Cypress is regarded as very gentle and suitable for all skin types. Avoid use during pregnancy.

Usage: Topical, Inhalation
Note: Middle-Base

Davana

Davana *(Artemisia pallens)* is used in aromatherapy as an agent to combat anxiety. It is a stimulant to the endocrine system. Davana is considered non-toxic and non-irritating.

Usage: Topical, Inhalation
Note: Base

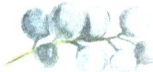

Dill

Dill *(Anethum graveolens)* is a stimulating, revitalizing, restoring, purifying, and balancing oil. Dill oil, when used aromatically, can help lessen stress and reduce anxious feelings. Its healing properties include carminative, galactagogue, and sedative. Dill Seed is non-toxic and non-irritating. Avoid use during pregnancy.

Usage: Oral, Topical, Inhalation
Note: Middle

Eucalyptus

Eucalyptus *(Eucalyptus radiata)* is used frequently in spas to lessen feelings of tension and promote relaxation. It is the perfect oil for sore muscles and joints. It is a very stimulating oil to the mind. Eucalyptus is considered toxic if taken internally. It is non-irritant and non-sensitive. Avoid if you have high blood pressure or epilepsy. It should be used in dilution. Please check with your healthcare provider before use during pregnancy.

Usage: Topical, Inhalation
Note: Top

Fennel

Fennel is credited with being carminative, depurative, diuretic, expectorant, laxative, and stimulant. It is believed to be invigorating, restoring, stimulating, and warming. Its therapeutic properties include aperitif, antiseptic, antispasmodic, emmenagogue, galactagogue, stomachic, splenic, tonic, and vermifuge. This oil may cause photosensitivity and contact dermatitis. Dilute well before use. Avoid use during pregnancy.

Usage: Oral, Topical, Inhalation
Note: Top-Middle

Frankincense

Frankincense *(Boswellia)* is highly prized in the aromatherapy industry as a potent anti-inflammatory with sedative properties. Frankincense oil can induce feelings of peace, satisfaction, and overall wellness. Frankincense helps to calm the body and mind. The therapeutic properties of Frankincense oil are carminative, cicatrisant, cytophylactic, emmenagogue, sedative, tonic, and vulnerary. Frankincense promotes relaxation to calm you and is known to send messages to the limbic system that help to reduce stress and improve mood. It can also help to reduce anxiety, pain, and inflammation. This oil is non-toxic, non-irritant, and non-sensitizing. Frankincense can be inhaled, applied topically, or ingested.

Usage: Oral, Topical, Inhalation
Note: Base

Galbanum

Galbanum *(Ferula gummosa Boiss)* is known for its respiratory treatment for asthma, bronchitis, and chronic coughs. It is also good for panic attacks and conditions of claustrophobia. This oil's properties include analgesic, antibacterial, antiviral, anti-inflammatory, antioxidant, antispasmodic, and an immunostimulant. Galbanum is non-toxic, non-irritant, and non-sensitizing. Use well-diluted. Avoid use during pregnancy.

Usage: Topical, Inhalation
Note: Top

Geranium

Geranium *(Pelargonium graveolens)* is a great all-over balancing effect on the body. It reduces edema and fluid retention, promotes circulation, and stimulates the lymphatic system. Inhaling Geranium oil can produce a calming, grounding effect. Geranium works well as a decent overall skin cleanser and makes an excellent oil for mature and troubled skin, bringing a radiant glow to your complexion. Geranium is well tolerated by most individuals, but since it helps in balancing the hormonal system, care must be taken during pregnancy. Avoid use during the first and second trimesters of pregnancy. Do not use if you have a history of estrogen-dependent cancer or are hypoglycemic.

Usage: Topical, Inhalation
Note: Middle

Grapefruit

Grapefruit *(Citrus × paradisi)* is spiritually uplifting, eases muscle fatigue and stiffness, relieves nervous exhaustion, and alleviates depression. It helps alleviate stress and lifts the spirit during dreary winters. Grapefruit is sometimes added to creams and lotions as a natural toner and cellulite treatment. Grapefruit's therapeutic properties are antidepressant, antiseptic, decongestant, diuretic, and tonic. It can cause photosensitivity.

Usage: Oral, Topical, Inhalation
Note: Top

Helichrysum

Helichrysum *(Helichrysum italicum)* is an effective oil for bruises, burns, cuts, dermatitis, eczema, irritated skin, and wounds. It supports the body through post-viral fatigue and recovery and can also be used to repair skin damaged by psoriasis, eczema, or ulceration. Helichrysum's therapeutic properties include cooling, anti-inflammatory, analgesic, antispasmodic, and as a tonic for the nervous system. This oil is non-toxic, non-irritating, and non-sensitizing. Please check with your healthcare provider before use during pregnancy.

Usage: Topical, Inhalation
Note: Base

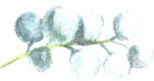

Ho Wood

Ho Wood *(Cinnamomum camphora)* has antidepressant, aphrodisiac, analgesic, anti-inflammatory, antispasmodic, sedative, immune support, tonic, and bactericidal properties. Ho Wood has become popular as a replacement for Rosewood because of its similar chemical qualities. It may irritate the skin. Avoid use during pregnancy.

Usage: Topical, Inhalation
Note: Middle

Jasmine

Jasmine *(Jasminun grandiflorum)* is a sensual, soothing, calming oil that promotes peace. It is important to note that all absolutes are extremely concentrated by nature. The complexity of the fragrance, particularly the rare and exotic notes, is well regarded as an aphrodisiac. However, it is also considered an antidepressant, antiseptic, cicatrisant, galactagogue, parturient, sedative, and antispasmodic. Jasmine has been known to assist with restless sleep. Use this oil to bring peace and relaxation to the body. Avoid use during the first and second trimesters of pregnancy.

Usage: Topical, Inhalation
Note: Base

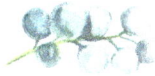

Juniper Berry

Juniper Berry *(Juniperus communis)* is a supportive, restoring, and tonic aid. It is considered purifying and clearing. When used aromatically, it can promote positive feelings and lessen feelings of stress. Juniper Berry's therapeutic properties are antispasmodic, carminative, depurative, diuretic, rubefacient, stimulating, stomachic, sudorific, vulnerary and tonic. Juniper Berry is non-irritating and non-sensitizing. Avoid use during pregnancy, and if you have a history of kidney disease or high blood pressure.

Usage: Topical, Inhalation
Note: Middle

Lavender

Lavender *(Lavandula angustifolia)* is predominately made up of alcohols and esters and has several therapeutic properties, many associated with relaxation. Lavender is the most popular essential oil, but be aware that several species, such as Spike Lavender *(Lavandula latifolia)* and Lavandin *(Lavandula x intermedia)*, have very similar properties but are not as sedating as true Lavender. Lavender is known to relieve restlessness and negative emotions. In one study, people who had inhaled Lavender oil the night before reported feeling more "vigorous" the next day. Lavender is known to calm anxiety and offers sedative effects. It can be suitable for anxious feelings due to its calming effects. Research revealed that a Lavender foot bath could improve blood flow and encourage changes in the autonomic nervous system often seen when people are relaxed. Applying some of this oil to the body diluted in a carrier oil before bed at night may also be effective. The therapeutic properties of Lavender essential oil are analgesic, anticonvulsant, antidepressant, antispasmodic, anti-inflammatory, carminative, cordial, hypotensive, nervine, sedative, and vulnerary. Lavender is non-toxic, non-irritating, and non-sensitizing. Do not use it during the first trimester of pregnancy.

Usage: Oral, Topical, Inhalation
Note: Middle

Lavandin

Lavandin *(Lavandula x intermedia)* properties include anticonvulsive, antidepressant, antiphlogistic, antispasmodic, antiviral, carminative, cordial, cytophylactic, and diuretic. Its calming scent reduces anxiety and promotes sleep. This oil is non-toxic, non-irritating, and non-sensitizing. Use caution if using during pregnancy.

Usage: Topical, Inhalation
Note: Middle

Lemon

Lemon *(Citrus limon)* is recognized due to its refreshing and cooling properties. This oil is uplifting and brightens one's mood. It is suitable for the circulatory system and aids blood flow, reducing blood pressure. Citral, myrcene, and limonene, all present in citrus oils, have been shown in some studies to lengthen sleep duration and relax muscles. Lemon's therapeutic properties are anti-anemic, carminative, hypotensive, and tonic. Lemon is non-toxic but could cause skin irritation for some. It is also phototoxic and should be avoided before exposure to direct sunlight.

Usage: Oral, Topical, Inhalation
Note: Top

Lemongrass

Lemongrass *(Cymbopogon citratus)* is known for its stimulating qualities and makes an excellent antidepressant. This essential oil promotes blood circulation by dilating the blood vessels, allowing uninterrupted blood flow. Lemongrass not only tones but fortifies the nervous system and can be used in the bath for soothing muscular nerves and pain with its potent analgesic and anti-inflammatory qualities. This oil relieves the symptoms of jet lag, helps with nervousness and anxiety, and clears headaches. The therapeutic properties of Lemongrass oil are analgesic, antidepressant, antipyretic, carminative, diuretic, febrifuge, nervine, nervous system sedative, and tonic. Avoid use with individuals with glaucoma. Use caution in prostatic hyperplasia and with skin hypersensitivity or damaged skin. Safe for topical and ingestion if appropriately diluted. It can be used topically, through diffusion/inhalation, and internally.

Usage: Oral, Topical, Inhalation
Note: Top

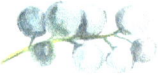

Lime

Lime *(Citrus × aurantiifolia)* has a crisp, refreshing citrus scent with uplifting and revitalizing properties that help with depression. Lime helps to relieve fatigue, apathy, and depression and is a great mood-lifter. The chemical constituents of Lime oil make it worthwhile for promoting emotional balance and well-being. This oil is also helpful for poor circulation and eliminating cellulite and obesity. The therapeutic properties of Lime are antiseptic, antiviral, astringent, aperitif, disinfectant, febrifuge, hemostatic, restorative, and tonic. Lime is considered phototoxic; users should avoid direct sunlight after application.

Usage: Oral, Topical, Inhalation
Note: Top

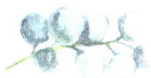

Linaloe Berry

Linaloe Berry *(Bursera delpechiana)* properties include anti-anxiety, antidepressant, antispasmodic, calming, sedative, and tonic. It promotes sleep and assists with pain caused by muscle soreness. This oil is considered non-irritating and non-sensitizing for most.

Usage: Topical, Inhalation
Note: Middle

Mandarin

Mandarin *(Citrus reticulata)* is often used to ease anxiety. This tangy oil increases circulation to the skin and reduces fluid retention. Mandarin therapeutic properties include sedative and tonic. Direct sunlight should be avoided after use, as it may be phototoxic.

Usage: Oral, Topical, Inhalation
Note: Top

Marjoram Sweet

Marjoram Sweet (Origanum marjorana) essential oil is recommended for helping with insomnia due to its calming and sedating action on the nervous system, which is known to lower blood pressure, ease nervous tension and hyperactivity, and soothe loneliness, grief, and rejection. Marjoram is a comforting oil that can be massaged into the affected area or added to a warm compress to ease discomfort. Marjoram is superb as a relaxant and is helpful for headaches, migraines, and insomnia. Marjoram's therapeutic properties are antispasmodic, anaphrodisiac, carminative, cordial, hypotensive, laxative, nervine, sedative, vasodilator, and vulnerary. Its sedative properties allow the body to heal, reduce inflammation and eliminate pain. Marjoram is generally non-toxic, non-irritating, and non-sensitizing.

Usage: Oral, Topical, Inhalation
Note: Middle

Melissa

Melissa *(Melissa officinalis)*, also called Lemon Balm, is well known for its antidepressant and uplifting properties. Its healing properties include antidepressant, antispasmodic, carminative, cordial, diaphoretic, emmenagogue, nervine, sedative, and tonic. Melissa has strong sedative qualities and treats emotional trauma and shock. This oil calms the nerves and comforts the soul. It is considered non-sensitizing and non-toxic. Please check with your healthcare provider before use during pregnancy.

Usage: Oral, Topical, Inhalation
Note: Middle-Top

Myrrh

Myrrh *(Commiphora myrrha)* is characterized as healing, tonic, stimulant, carminative, diaphoretic, bitter, circulatory stimulant, and antispasmodic. This oil is well known for its spiritual aspects but is also suitable for treating female complaints. Myrrh oil can help increase spiritual awareness and promote a creative, inspiring, energetic mood. Myrrh is calming to the spirit and is frequently used for meditation. Myrrh can be toxic in high concentrations and should not be used during pregnancy.

Usage: Topical, Inhalation
Note: Base

Neroli

Neroli *(Citrus aurantium amara)* is used for its relaxing and slightly hypnotic effects, and it can also help with lucid dreaming and creativity. It aids restful sleep due to its soothing qualities as a natural tranquilizer. One study found that Neroli oil, in combination with Lavender and Chamomile oil, was effective in reducing anxiety, increasing sleep, and stabilizing blood pressure. Neroli is also known to help relieve muscle spasms and heart palpitations. Neroli's therapeutic properties are antidepressant, antispasmodic, aphrodisiac, carminative, cytophylactic, cordial, sedative, and tonic. This oil is non-toxic and non-sensitizing.

Usage: Topical, Inhalation
Note: Middle-Top

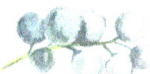

Opoponax

Opoponax *(Commiphora erythraea)*, also known as Sweet Myrrh, has anti-anxiety, calming, carminative, sedative, tonic, and vulnerable properties. This oil is helpful for menopause. It is also beneficial for relaxing muscles, reducing stress, and treating anxiety. It may be phototoxic; therefore, avoid direct sunlight for 12 hours. Avoid use during pregnancy.

Usage: Topical, Inhalation
Note: Base

Orange, Bitter

Orange, Bitter *(Citrus × aurantium)* is remarkably similar to Sweet Orange in therapeutic properties as an antidepressant, anti-inflammatory, antispasmodic, aphrodisiac, bactericidal, carminative, stomachic, cordial, deodorant, digestive, fungicidal, stimulant for the nervous system, and a tonic for the circulatory system. Orange Bitter essential oil is effective in treating stress. It is considered phototoxic, so exposure to sunlight should be avoided after use. Avoid use during pregnancy.

Usage: Topical, Inhalation
Note: Top

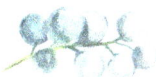

Orange, Sweet

Orange, Sweet *(Citrus × sinensis)* works as an antidepressant, antiseptic, antispasmodic, aphrodisiac, carminative, deodorant, stimulant (nervous), and tonic for the cardiac and circulatory systems. It helps with stress and uplifts, calming digestive problems and eliminating toxins. It stimulates the lymphatic system and supports collagen formation in the skin. It is considered phototoxic; therefore, exposure to sunlight should be avoided.

Usage: Oral, Topical, Inhalation
Note: Top

Palo Santo

Palo Santo *(Bursera graveolens)* is excellent for massage therapy to relieve pain and inflammation of the muscles and joints. This oil is also beneficial for panic attacks, anxiety, headaches, migraines, concentration, and focus. Palo Santo's properties include antispasmodic, decongestant, expectorant, and a nervous system tonic. This oil may cause skin irritation. Avoid use during pregnancy.

Usage: Topical, Inhalation
Note: Top

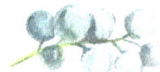

Patchouli

Patchouli *(Pogostemon cablin)* is beneficial for combating nervous disorders and nausea and treating depression. This oil's therapeutic properties include antidepressant, aphrodisiac, nervine, prophylactic, stimulating, and tonic agent. As a sedative oil, it allows the body to relax and rest, allowing healing to begin. It is considered a grounding oil and helps to balance emotions. It may interact with aspirin, blood pressure, antiplatelet, and anticoagulant medications and increase the risk of bleeding among people with bleeding disorders.

Usage: Oral, Topical, Inhalation
Note: Base

Pepper, Black

Pepper, Black *(Piper nigrum)* is used to treat pain, rheumatism, poor circulation, exhaustion, and muscular aches and to stimulate the appetite. Black Pepper is a potent anti-inflammatory agent. Its properties include analgesic, antiseptic, antispasmodic, anti-toxic, aphrodisiac, antiemetic, antiviral, digestive, diuretic, expectorant, febrifuge, rubefacient, and warming. This oil may irritate sensitive skin and overstimulate the kidneys if used too much.

Usage: Oral, Topical, Inhalation
Note: Middle-Base

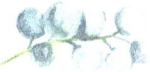

Peppermint

Peppermint *(Mentha × piperita)* has long been credited as being useful in combating stomach ailments and soothing the digestive system. Its energizing effect is significant for invigorating the spirit and one's mood. It's great for headaches, travel sickness, and jet lag. Its properties include antifungal, antiseptic, antispasmodic, astringent, anti-inflammatory, analgesic, carminative, febrifuge, decongestant, expectorant, and stimulating to the circulatory and immune systems. Peppermint can be sensitizing due to its menthol content. Do not use it if you have cardiac fibrillation. Please check with your healthcare provider regarding use during pregnancy. Avoid if you have a history of high blood pressure.

Usage: Oral, Topical, Inhalation
Note: Top-Middle

Petitgrain

Petitgrain *(Citrus × aurantium)* is believed to have uplifting properties and is used for calming anger and stress. Petitgrain is valued for its calming qualities, making it a favorite for insomnia. This oil's properties include antidepressant, stimulant, tonic, and sedative for the nervous system. The aroma of Petitgrain oil can help ease feelings of tension and promote calmness. Petitgrain is generally considered non-toxic, non-irritant, and non-sensitizing.

Usage: Oral, Topical, Inhalation
Note: Top

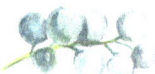

Rosalina

Rosalina *(Melaleuca ericifolia)* is well known for its spasmolytic and anticonvulsant properties. Rosalina has properties that help to relax and calm individuals who may be stressed deeply. It is helpful for insomnia and other sleep disorders. Rosalina's therapeutic properties include analgesic and anti-anxiety. Avoid use during pregnancy.

Usage: Topical, Inhalation
Note: Middle

Rose Geranium

Rose Geranium *(Pelargonium graveolens)* has the ability to both uplift and sedate. It is considered a wonder oil for emotions and balances the hormonal system. Rose Geranium is non-toxic, non-irritant, and generally non-sensitizing, though it can cause sensitivity in some people. Its therapeutic properties include being an antidepressant and sedative. Avoid use during pregnancy.

Usage: Oral, Topical, Inhalation
Note: Middle

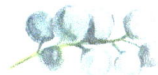

Rose

Rose *(Rosa × damascena)* is an uplifting aphrodisiac and is excellent for meditation. Rose oil treats depression, grief, anger, and other unpleasant emotions. It supports the heart and is considered one of the most amazing remedies for irritability. The therapeutic properties of Rose are antidepressant, antiphlogistic, aphrodisiac, nervous system sedative, and a tonic for the heart. Avoid use during the first trimester of pregnancy.

Usage: Oral, Topical, Inhalation
Note: Base

Rosemary

Rosemary *(Rosemarinus officinalis)* is a warming oil that improves circulation and helps overcome mental fatigue and sluggishness by stimulating and strengthening the entire nervous system. It also enhances mental clarity while aiding alertness and concentration. It is also beneficial to use in stressful conditions. Rosemary is generally non-toxic and non-sensitizing but unsuitable for people with epilepsy or high blood pressure. Rosemary's therapeutic properties are analgesic, anti-inflammatory, anti-rheumatic, antiseptic, astringent, antispasmodic, antiviral, decongestant, diuretic, expectorant, restorative, and stimulant. Avoid use during pregnancy.

Usage: Oral, Topical, Inhalation
Note: Middle

Rosewood

Rosewood *(Dalbergia latifolia)* is credited as being a stimulant, tonic, antidepressant, sedative, and aphrodisiac. It is also regarded as a general balancer of emotions. Rosewood is rich in linalool. It is a possible irritant to sensitive skin. Avoid use during pregnancy.

Usage: Topical, Inhalation
Note: Base

Sage

Sage *(Salvia officinalis)* is believed to calm the nerves and assist with grief and depression, female sterility, and menopausal problems. The therapeutic properties of Sage oil are anti-inflammatory, antibacterial, antiseptic, antispasmodic, astringent, digestive, diuretic, emmenagogue, febrifuge, hypertensive, laxative, stomachic, and tonic. It should not be used by persons with epilepsy or high blood pressure. Use in low concentration.

Usage: Oral, Topical, Inhalation
Note: Top-Middle

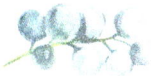

Sandalwood

Sandalwood *(Santalum album)* is known to create an exotic, sensual mood with a reputation as an aphrodisiac. Its sedative effect allows the body to relax and heal. Sandalwood is used to help combat mood disturbances and stress. Santalol, a major component of sandalwood oil, has been found to have a depressive effect on the central nervous system, enabling users to get more sleep. Sandalwood's therapeutic properties include being a sedative and tonic. Sandalwood can aid in relaxation and calm anxiety. It is also known to have soothing effects. Sandalwood is considered non-toxic, non-irritant, and non-sensitizing.

Usage: Oral, Topical, Inhalation
Note: Base

Spearmint

Spearmint *(Mentha spicata)* is a local or topical anesthetic with stimulant and restorative properties. Spearmint is an uplifting oil, making it ideal for alleviating fatigue and depression. The fresh aroma of Spearmint oil uplifts mood while promoting a sense of focus. Spearmint may irritate mucous membranes. Please check with your healthcare provider before use during the first trimester of pregnancy.

Usage: Oral, Topical, Inhalation
Note: Top

Spikenard

Spikenard *(Nardostachys jatamansi)* is used by aromatherapists because it brings peaceful tranquility. This oil's therapeutic properties include being a sedative and tonic. It is a good oil for grounding emotions. Spikenard should be avoided during pregnancy.

Usage: Oral, Topical, Inhalation
Note: Base

Spruce

Spruce *(Picea pungens)* is used in baths for tired muscles, room sprays, detergents, and cough and cold preparations. Its therapeutic properties include anti-inflammatory, anti-rheumatic, antispasmodic, antiseptic, decongestant, diuretic, rubefacient, and warming. At low doses, it is non-toxic, non-irritating, and non-sensitizing.

Usage: Topical, Inhalation
Note: Middle

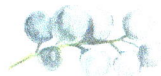

Tangerine

Tangerine *(Citrus reticulata)* is a refreshing and rejuvenating oil that clears the mind and helps eliminate emotional confusion. Tangerine is genuinely comforting and soothing and brings happiness. Its healing properties include antispasmodic, carminative, digestive stimulant, diuretic, sedative, stimulant for the lymphatic system, and tonic agent. Like other essential oils in the citrus family, Tangerine can be phototoxic. The skin should not be exposed to sunlight after a treatment. This oil should be diluted well before use on the skin.

Usage: Oral, Topical, Inhalation
Note: Top

Tea Tree

Tea Tree *(Melaleuca alternifolia)* is best known as a powerful immune stimulant. It helps fight all three categories of infectious organisms: bacterial, viral, and fungal. It clears up pimples and reduces their reoccurrence due to its antimicrobial and anti-inflammatory power. Tea Tree's therapeutic properties are antimicrobial, antiseptic, antiviral, balsamic, bactericide, cicatrisant, expectorant, fungicidal, insecticide, stimulant and sudorific. Tea Tree may cause dermal sensitization in some people. Do not take it internally.

Usage: Topical, Inhalation
Note: Top

Thyme

Thyme *(Thymus vulgaris)* is considered a stimulating, uplifting, and reviving oil. The therapeutic properties of Thyme oil are anti-rheumatic, antispasmodic, bechic, cardiac, carminative, cicatrisant, diuretic, emmenagogue, expectorant, hypertensive, stimulant, and tonic. It helps with mental concentration. Thyme's warming qualities make it great for rheumatism, sciatica, arthritis, and gout. Red Thyme and White Thyme are used in aromatherapy; please dilute properly as it is a potential skin irritant. Avoid use during pregnancy.

Usage: Oral, Topical, Inhalation
Note: Middle-Top

Verbena, Lemon

Verbena, Lemon *(Aloysia citrodora)* is considered an aphrodisiac, sedative, and tonic. Verbena soothes the circulatory system and calms heart palpitations. Its calming action helps to banish depression and uplift the spirit. This oil assists with nervous conditions, especially those that manifest as digestive complaints. Verbena softens the skin and helps to reduce puffiness.

Usage: Topical, Inhalation
Note: Top

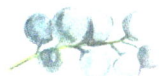

Valerian

Valerian *(Valeriana officinalis)* is used in combating nervousness, restlessness, tension, agitation, panic attacks, and headaches resulting from nervous tension. It has been used for heart palpitations and has gained popularity as a natural alternative to commercially available sedatives. The therapeutic properties of Valerian include being a carminative, hypnotic, hypotensive, regulator, and sedative. It has possible skin-sensitizing properties, though it is non-toxic and non-irritating at low doses. Avoid use during pregnancy and with children. Valerian has been shown to reduce anxiety. It is calming to the nervous system and helps with restlessness.

Usage: Oral, Topical, Inhalation
Note: Base

Vetiver

Vetiver *(Chrysopogon zizanioides)* is profoundly relaxing and comforting. Its calming and soothing effect helps to dispel irritability, anger, and hysteria while having a balancing effect on the hormonal system. It is relaxing to the nervous system and helps with overstimulation. Vetiver oil's therapeutic properties are aphrodisiac, cicatrisant, nervine, sedative, tonic, and vulnerary. There is no known toxicity.

Usage: Oral, Topical, Inhalation
Note: Base

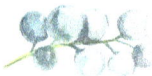

Violet Leaf

Violet Leaf *(Viola)* is known for being a relaxing and soothing oil. It can be used for stress, headaches, nervousness, and insomnia. This oil is considered non-toxic and non-irritating but may cause sensitization in some individuals.

Usage: Topical, Inhalation
Note: Base-Middle

Wintergreen

Wintergreen *(Gaultheria procumbens)* serves as a stimulant, emmenagogue, and anti-rheumatic. It is beneficial in rheumatic conditions and helps with muscular pains, especially for athletes. Avoid use during pregnancy. Safety with young children, nursing women, or those with severe liver or kidney disease is unknown.

Usage: Topical, Inhalation
Note: Middle

White Fir

White Fir *(Abies concolor)* is used for encouragement and empowerment. White Fir combats negative feelings and enables you to stand tall. Its properties include anti-arthritic, antiseptic, expectorant, analgesic, anti-catarrhal, and stimulant. This oil may cause possible skin sensitivity. If pregnant, consult your physician before use.

Usage: Topical, Inhalation
Note: Middle

Ylang Ylang

Ylang Ylang *(Cananga odorata)* assists with problems such as rapid breathing, heartbeat, and nervous conditions due to its calming effect. The therapeutic properties of Ylang Ylang are antidepressant, aphrodisiac, hypotensive, nervine, and sedative. Ylang Ylang helps balance both sides of the brain and aid in the processing and releasing of negative emotions like anger. Ylang Ylang oil can be combined with Bergamot oil to help reduce blood pressure, pulse, stress, anxiety, and cortisol. Ylang Ylang is also a sedative and can help relieve anxiety. Ylang Ylang may cause sensitivity in some people, and excessive use may lead to headaches and nausea. This oil is not recommended if you have low blood pressure. Ylang Ylang is an excellent oil for quieting the mind if you find your mind racing through the day's activities and are struggling to settle it.

Usage: Oral, Topical, Inhalation
Note: Base

CHAPTER 7

COMMON EMOTIONS AND ESSENTIAL OILS

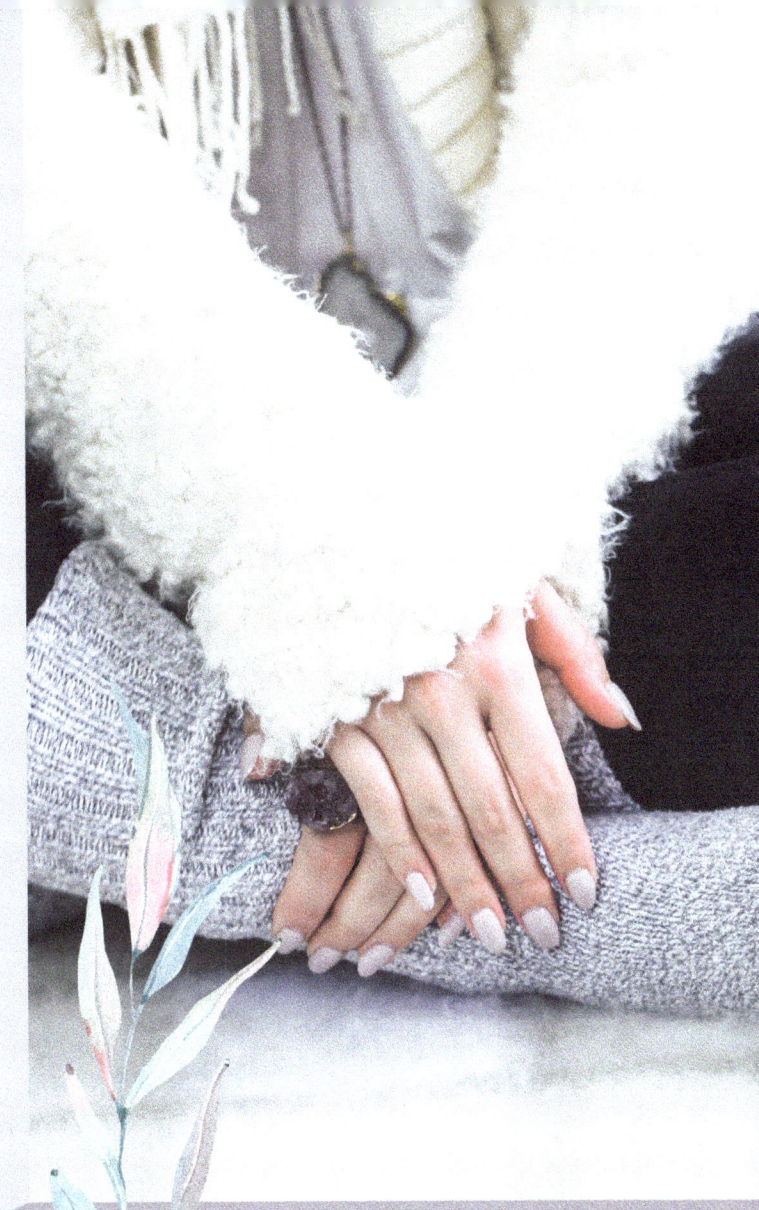

Listed below are some of the most common emotions you may experience at one time or another—some feelings you may want to suppress, others you may want to enhance with the help of essential oils.

ANGER

Anger is a powerful emotion characterized by frustration, unhappiness, or rage. Use these oils to help alleviate this emotion.

TOP	MIDDLE	BASE
Bergamot	Chamomile, Roman	Jasmine
Orange	Marjoram	Patchouli
Petitgrain	Neroli	Rose
	Palmarosa	Vetiver
	Rosemary	Ylang Ylang

AGGRESSION

Aggression is a hostile feeling which could be accompanied by violent behavior or attitudes toward another person or thing. Try one of these oils for relief.

TOP	MIDDLE	BASE
Bergamot	Chamomile, Roman	Ylang Ylang
Lemon	Juniper Berry	
	Marjoram	
	Rosemary	

ANXIETY

Anxiety is a feeling of apprehension, uneasiness, or discomfort, typically concerning an upcoming event or situation with an uncertain outcome. Use one of these oils to relieve the discomfort of this emotion.

TOP	MIDDLE	BASE
Basil	Ambrette Seed	Benzoin
Bergamot	Chamomile, Roman	Cedarwood
Clary Sage	Geranium	Frankincense
Mandarin	Hyssop	Jasmine
Orange	Juniper Berry	Patchouli
Peppermint	Lavender	Rose
	Marjoram	Sandalwood
	Melissa	Vetiver
	Neroli	Valerian
	Spruce	Ylang Ylang

CALM

Calm is a feeling of tranquil and quiet; soothing. Use one of these oils to soothe your soul.

TOP	MIDDLE	BASE
Clary Sage	Blue Tansy	Balsam
Galbanum	Fir	Cistus Labdanum
Palo Santo	Geranium	Helichrysum
Petitgrain	Ho Wood	Jasmine
Lemon Verbena	Juniper Berry	Myrrh
	Lavandin	Opoponax

	Lavender	Patchouli
	Linaloe Berry	Rose
	Marjoram	Rosewood
	Palmarosa	Sandalwood
	Pine	Spikenard
	Rosalina	Wormwood
	Thyme	
	Yarrow	

CONFIDENCE

Confidence is a feeling of self-assurance from one's appreciation of one's abilities or qualities. Use one of these oils to support yourself when lacking confidence.

TOP	MIDDLE	BASE
Bay Laurel	Cypress	Jasmine
Bergamot	Rosemary	
Grapefruit		
Orange		

DEPRESSION

Depression is a feeling of persistent sadness. It also manifests as a lack of interest or pleasure in previously rewarding or enjoyable activities. Use one of these essential oils to lift your spirits.

TOP	MIDDLE	BASE
Bergamot	Chamomile, Roman	Frankincense
Clary Sage	Geranium	Helichrysum
Grapefruit	Lavender	Jasmine

Lemon	Neroli	Rose
Mandarin		Sandalwood
Orange		Ylang Ylang

DISAPPOINTMENT

Disappointment is sadness or displeasure caused by the nonfulfillment of one's hopes or expectations. Try one or more of these essential oils to renew your hope for the future.

TOP	MIDDLE	BASE
Bay Laurel	Cypress	Frankincense
Bergamot	Rosemary	Jasmine
Orange		Rose

FATIGUE OR EXHAUSTION

Fatigue is extreme tiredness resulting from mental or physical exertion or illness. Try one of these oils to help alleviate exhaustion and renew your strength.

TOP	MIDDLE	BASE
Basil	Black Pepper	Frankincense
Bergamot	Clary Sage	Ginger
Coriander	Cinnamon	Helichrysum
Eucalyptus	Cypress	Jasmine
Grapefruit	Juniper Berry	Patchouli
Lemon	Palmarosa	Sandalwood
Orange	Peppermint	Vetiver
	Rosemary	Ylang Ylang

FEAR

Fear is an unpleasant emotion caused by the belief that someone or something is dangerous, likely to cause pain or a threat. Try one or more of these oils to help you feel safe and overcome fear.

TOP	MIDDLE	BASE
Bergamot	Chamomile	Cedarwood
Clary Sage	Neroli	Frankincense
Fennel	Thyme	Ginger
Grapefruit		Jasmine
Lemon		Patchouli
Orange		Sandalwood

GRIEF OR SADNESS

Sadness or grief is deep sorrow, especially caused by someone's death. Use one or more of these oils to help restore comfort and joy in your heart.

TOP	MIDDLE	BASE
Bergamot	Chamomile	Benzoin
	Cypress	Frankincense
	Marjoram	Helichrysum
	Neroli	Jasmine
		Rose
		Rosewood
		Sandalwood
		Vetiver

HAPPINESS OR CONTENTMENT

Contentment is a state of happiness and satisfaction. Use one or more of these oils when your soul longs for brighter and happier days.

TOP	MIDDLE	BASE
Bergamot	Geranium	Frankincense
Grapefruit	Neroli	Rose
Lemon		Sandalwood
Orange		Ylang Ylang

HYSTERIA

Hysteria is an exaggerated or uncontrollable emotion or excitement—no need to panic when you have one of these essential oils around. Grab a bottle and sniff for instant relief.

TOP	MIDDLE	BASE
Orange	Chamomile, Roman	Frankincense
Tea Tree	Lavender	Valerian
	Neroli	

IMPATIENCE

Impatience is the tendency to be impatient, irritable, or restless. These oils can help you regain composure.

TOP	MIDDLE	BASE
Clary Sage	Chamomile, Roman	Frankincense
	Lavender	

INDECISIVENESS

Can't seem to make up your mind? Try one of these oils when you struggle making up your mind or can't seem to make decisions quickly and effectively.

TOP	MIDDLE	BASE
Basil	Cypress	Jasmine
Clary Sage	Peppermint	Patchouli

INSECURITY

When uncertainty or anxiety about oneself creeps in, try one of these essential oils.

TOP	MIDDLE	BASE
Bergamot	Chamomile, Roman	Cedarwood
	Lavender	Frankincense
		Jasmine
		Sandalwood
		Vetiver

IRRITABILITY

Are you bordering on blowing your stack? Why not try one of these essential oils to help you be rational about the situation?

TOP	MIDDLE	BASE
Mandarin	Chamomile, Roman	Sandalwood
	Lavender	
	Neroli	

JEALOUSY

When the green-eyed monster gets the best of you, grab one of these essential oils to remind you how great you are.

TOP	MIDDLE	BASE
		Jasmine
		Rose
		Ylang Ylang

LONELINESS

Feeling alone or left behind? During a moment of solitude, diffuse one of these essential oils.

TOP	MIDDLE	BASE
Bergamot	Chamomile, Roman	Benzoin
Clary Sage	Marjoram	Frankincense
		Helichrysum
		Rose

MEMORY OR CONCENTRATION

Trouble recalling something? Or can't seem to focus your attention on the task at hand? Try one of these oils.

TOP	MIDDLE	BASE
Basil	Cypress	
Lemon	Hyssop	
Peppermint	Rosemary	

NERVOUSNESS

Are you shaking in your boots? No need to suffer. Grab one of these oils and take a deep breath or two.

TOP	MIDDLE	BASE
Clary Sage	Chamomile, Roman	Frankincense
Coriander	Lavender	Vetiver
Orange	Neroli	Ylang Ylang

PANIC OR PANIC ATTACKS

Panic attacks are sudden feelings of acute and disabling anxiety. You can stop panic attacks dead in their tracks with one of these essential oils in a personal inhaler for instant relief.

TOP	MIDDLE	BASE
Clary Sage	Chamomile, Roman	Frankincense
	Geranium	Helichrysum
	Juniper Berry	Jasmine
	Lavender	Rose
	Neroli	Ylang Ylang

SHOCK

Shock strikes when a sudden upsetting, or surprising event or experience happens. Be ready with one of these essential oils nearby.

TOP	MIDDLE	BASE
Tea Tree	Lavender	Rose
	Neroli	Valerian

SHYNESS

Shyness can make you feel uncomfortable, self-conscious, nervous, bashful, timid, or insecure around others. Take control of the situation with one of these essential oils. Be bold.

TOP	MIDDLE	BASE
Peppermint	Black Pepper	Jasmine
	Ginger	Patchouli
	Neroli	Rose
		Ylang Ylang

STRESS

Stress is an emotion that results from an event or thought that causes pressure. Try any of the following essential oils to help you in your hour of need.

TOP	MIDDLE	BASE
Bergamot	Chamomile, Roman	Benzoin
Clary Sage	Geranium	Cedarwood
Grapefruit	Lavender	Frankincense
Mandarin	Marjoram	Jasmine
Petitgrain	Melissa	Patchouli
	Neroli	Rose
	Rosemary	Sandalwood
		Vetiver
		Ylang Ylang

TENSION

Tension is mental or emotional strain—no need to suffer when you have one of these essential oils nearby.

TOP	MIDDLE	BASE
Clary Sage	Chamomile, Roman	Frankincense
Lemon	Cypress	Jasmine
Orange	Geranium	Rose
	Lavender	Rosewood
	Marjoram	Sandalwood
	Neroli	Ylang Ylang

CHAPTER 8

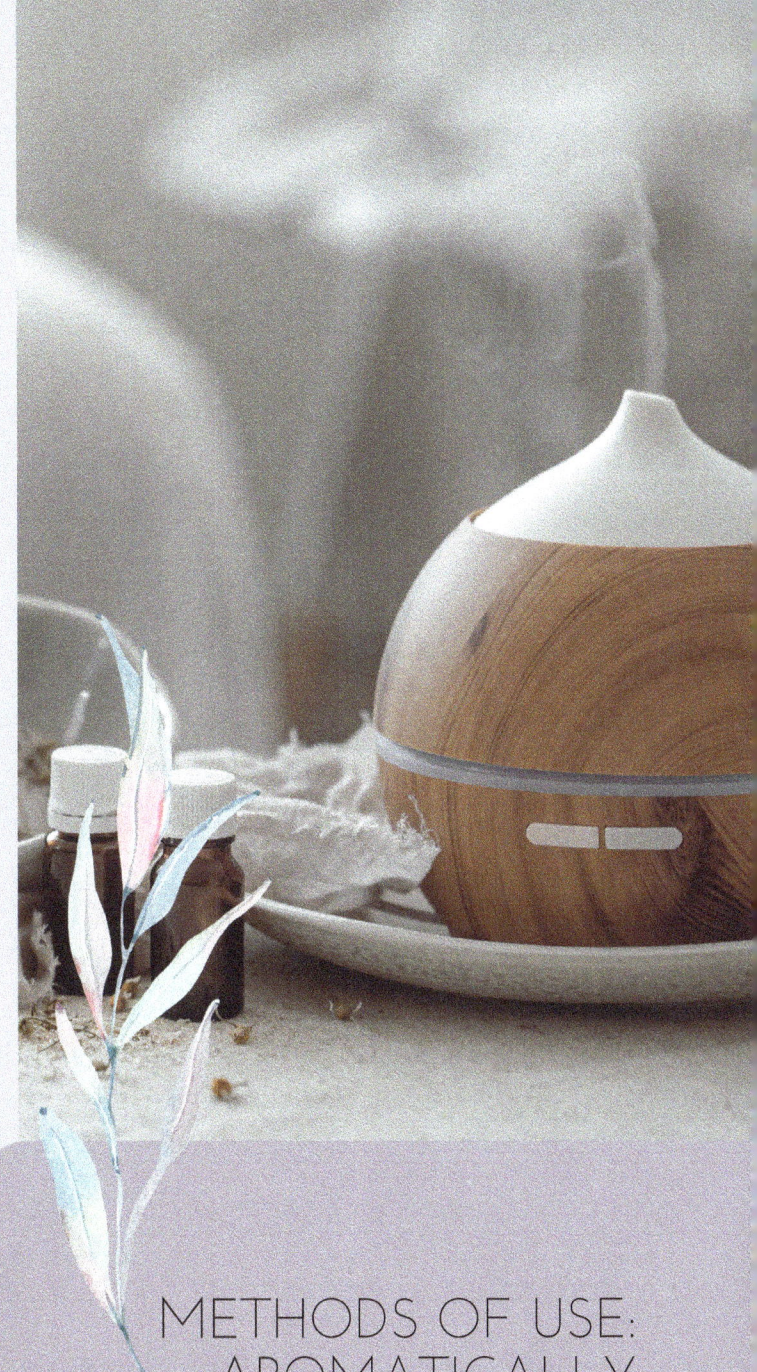

METHODS OF USE: AROMATICALLY

Several options are available for healing emotions with essential oils. Various mechanisms can be used to deliver essential oils. Typical routes of administration include inhalation, topical, and ingestion. Regardless of which route of administration is used, the essential oils have to travel to the site of action with either the help of blood, nerves, or oxygen (when the inhalation route is used). Combining these three approaches will ensure success.

INHALATION

Inhalation is one of the most natural methods of use and is considered the most direct pathway for an aromatic blend or essence. When inhaled, fragrant vapors enter the lungs and are instantly released into the bloodstream for delivery to every cell in the body. Scientific research shows that essential oils can remain in a person's bloodstream for up to 4-6 hours, depending on the essential oil.

Essential oils that are adequately diffused are known to improve mental clarity, enhance or calm emotions, and increase feelings of well-being. If a diffuser is not available, making a room spray, personal inhaler, or placing a few drops on a tissue to inhale will suffice. All are very effective ways to benefit from the therapeutic properties of essential oils. For inhalation, use intermittent exposure (not more than 15 minutes in an hour).

Inhalation of essential oil vapors triggers the olfactory bulb, which immediately sends a neurochemical signal to neuro-receptors. For example, smelling Lavender essential oil triggers the release of serotonin from the raphe nucleus in the brain and produces a calmative effect. Essential oils can easily be absorbed via inhalation and enter the bloodstream to deliver healing constituents throughout the body. Inhalation presents the least amount of risk for most individuals.

INHALATION METHODS FOR EMOTIONS

Diffuser – Try adding essential oil or a blend of choice to a diffuser. Use a nebulizer to diffuse your selection of oils for an hour three times a day. You may want to use one specific essential oil (with no carrier oil added). Or, you may blend a combination of essential oils. Place 10-12 essential oil into a diffuser and use as needed. Limit the diffusion of new oils to 10 minutes each day, increasing the time until the desired effects are reached. Adjust times for different-sized rooms and the strength of each fragrance.

Cup Hands – Place 2-3 drops of your chosen essential oil in your hand and rub your palms together. Cup hands over your nose and inhale deeply.

Personal Inhaler – Add 1-2 drops of essential oil to a tissue and carry it with you to smell throughout the day, or add several drops of pure essential oil to a pocket diffuser and use it 2-3 times daily.

Room Spray – Spritz your pillow and bedsheets with a relaxing fragrance before bed.

Smelling Salts - In a small tub or 10 ml (1/3 oz.) glass bottle, add 30 drops of the essential oil blend and fill the remainder of the bottle with either fine or coarse sea salt. Waft the bottle under your nose while taking deep inhalations whenever you feel the need to relax your emotions.

Shower Steamers – Make these ahead and drop them in a hot shower or bath to relax. You can also add a few drops of a relaxing essential oil to Epsom salts for a nice bedtime bath!

Cotton Ball – Add a few drops to a tissue or cotton ball and tuck it inside your pillowcase.

Bottle – Open the bottle and take a sniff several times before going to sleep.

Humidifier/Vaporizer – Place ten drops of essential oil undiluted in a humidifier or vaporizer to diffuse into the air.

DIFFUSER BLENDS

Pleasant, relaxing aromas used in a diffuser are one of the most effective ways to improve a mood. The diffuser transforms the oil into a fine mist of oil droplets which disperse the scent throughout the air. This enables you to enjoy its pleasing aroma for an extended time, making it the most convenient way to use essential oils for healing emotions.

HOW TO CHOOSE AN ESSENTIAL OIL DIFFUSER

There are plenty of essential oil diffusers to choose from. Before buying one, evaluate your needs to determine which model will serve you best. Be sure the diffuser doesn't heat the oil as this may change its molecular structure, rendering it less potent and effective (glass nebulizer, waterless is best).

USING AN ESSENTIAL OIL DIFFUSER SAFELY

If you have other health conditions, you may want to consult with a certified aromatherapist before using essential oils aromatically to improve sleep. Essential oils can be highly potent, and reactions will differ from person to person.

BLENDING ESSENTIAL OILS

Combining several essential oils in one diffuser is one way to enjoy the benefits of essential oil diffusion. Blending your diffuser blend creates a new aroma that is unique and different. The number of combinations you can make are limitless, but it might be difficult to know which oils pair well with others and which don't. For best results, follow the instructions below to learn how to make essential oil blends at home.

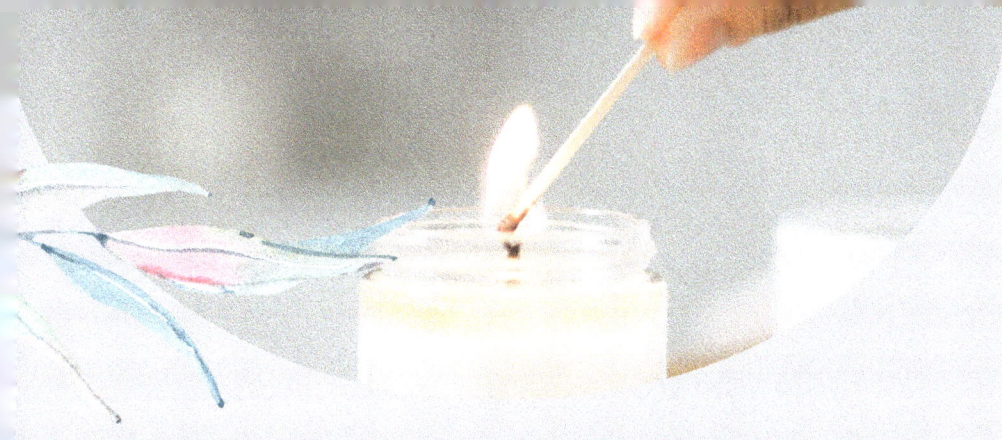

TIPS FOR MAKING A GOOD DIFFUSER BLEND

01 Determine the desired effect you want from the diffuser blend. The oil you use will determine the feeling you want to experience, such as relaxing, calming, or invigorating.

Are you trying to create a calming environment? Once you determine the desired outcome, choosing oils that complement one another will be easier.

02 Choose a group of oils with similar properties to help you achieve your desired effect. If you want a relaxing diffuser blend, choose oils known for calmness and serenity, like Lavender. Choose oils with stimulating properties like Peppermint or Lemon if you want an energizing effect.

03 Once you have decided on the oils you want to use, you can begin pairing them together.

PAIRING SIMILAR OILS

When creating a unique diffuser blend, combine essential oils of the same type or category. For example, citrus oils like Bergamot, Lemon, and Grapefruit fall within the same category, so you know they will pair well together.

PAIRING DIFFERENT OILS

When you want to add variety to your essential oil blends, you can pair oils from different categories together for various new aromas. As you blend oils from different categories, you can end up with a unique blend that showcases the best attributes of each oil.

PAIRING OILS FROM DIFFERENT CATEGORIES

- Floral oils blend well with spicy, woody, and citrus oils
- Spicy oils blend well with citrus, woody, and floral oils
- Citrus oils blend well with woody, floral, spicy, and mint oils
- Herbaceous essential oils blend well with mint and woody oils
- Mint essential oils blend well with woody, earthy, herbaceous, and citrus oils

PERSONAL INHALERS

Essential oil inhalers are an excellent way to enjoy the perks of essential oils even when you're not at home or unable to use a diffuser. They're portable, practical, and discreet. This blending and recipe guide will show you how to make your inhaler blends.

What You Will Need:

Inhaler apparatus
Label
Essential oils for the blend you choose
Fractionated coconut oil (optional)
Tiny bowl
Pipette
Tweezers
Surgical/Exam gloves

Plastic inhalers are typically made of four parts: a cover, a wick, a wick enclosure, and a cap. Aluminum inhalers are generally made of a glass vial, a wick, an aluminum screw-on top with air holes, an outer aluminum enclosure, and an aluminum cap.

Many diffuser blends can be used as inspiration for creating inhaler blends. However, thoroughly research the safety precautions for each essential oil you plan to use in your blend and limit the number of drops to fifteen or less per inhaler.

WHAT TO DO FOR PLASTIC INHALER ASSEMBLY:

1. Mix the essential oils for your chosen blend in a tiny bowl.
2. If you prefer the inhaler not to be intensely aromatic, add approximately 5-15 drops of fractionated coconut oil into your essential oil blend to weaken the scent. You will need to experiment with the dilution to achieve your desired aromatic strength.
3. Place the wick in the bowl.
4. Using your tweezers, rotate the wick around to completely absorb the essential oil blend.
5. Once the wick is saturated with the oil, use the tweezers to pick it up and place it in the wick enclosure (the part with a hole at the top).
6. Secure the end cap or butt onto the cotton wick opening.
7. Screw the outer cover onto the wick opening.
8. Label your inhaler.
9. Keep the lid/cover on the inhaler when you are not using it.

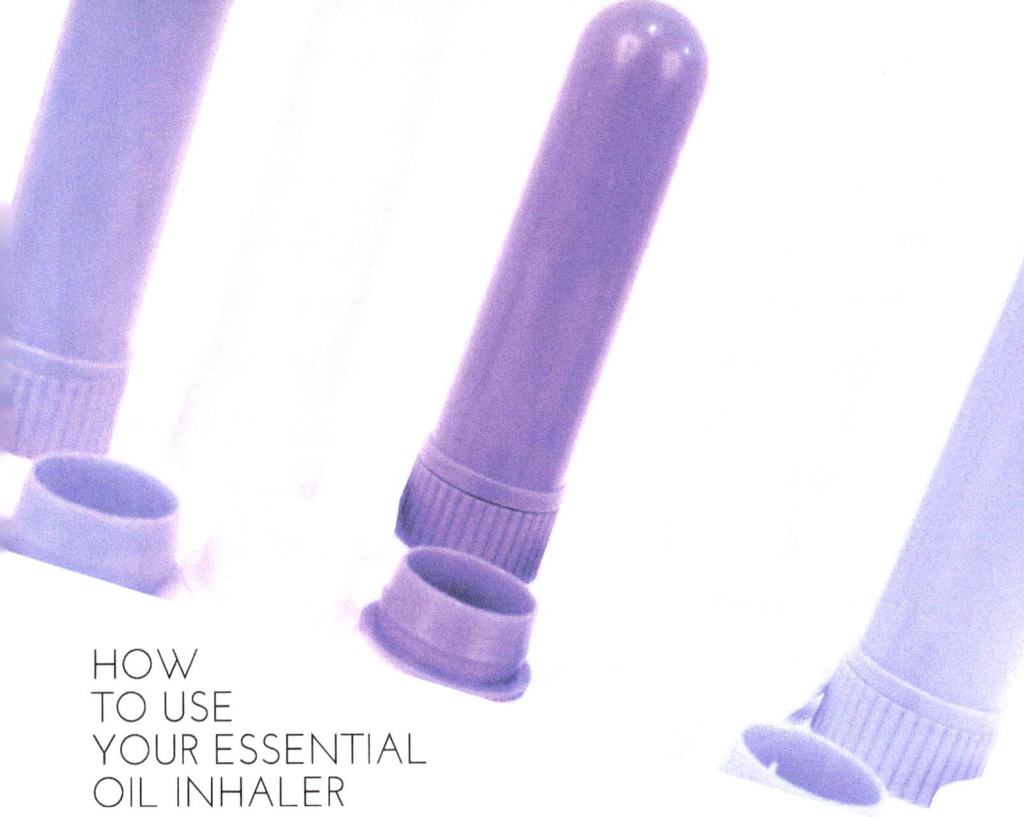

HOW TO USE YOUR ESSENTIAL OIL INHALER

- Remove the cap from your essential oil inhaler.
- Raise it to one nostril, ensuring that the tip of the inhaler does not come into direct contact with your nose (or other skin).
- Inhale as deeply as is comfortable.
- Repeat with the other nostril.
- Close the cap.
- If you experience any adverse reactions, discontinue using your inhaler immediately.

Keep in mind everyone is different. Check the safety information to ensure the oil is appropriate for personal use. The essential oil blends suggested in this book are for use by healthy adults with no serious underlying medical issues. Cut the number of drops in half for children under six.

ROOM SPRAY

A room spray is a type of diffusion that quickly releases a concentrated amount of oil into the air. If hydrosol is unavailable, you will use approximately 30-40 drops of essential oil in hydrosol or mineral water and vodka. Use as needed to create a unique atmosphere.

To ensure the essential oils disperse throughout the hydrosol or another water-based carrier (and stay mixed), you will need to add a product called "Solubol," an all-natural dispersant. If you do not have this, you may substitute aloe vera or glycerin in its place.

Room sprays are great for changing the mood of a room. You may choose any fragrant hydrosol or floral water for your base. Some of the best ones for creating a pleasant, soothing atmosphere include Lavender and Roman Chamomile. If you want a more romantic feel for your space, you may wish to use Ylang Ylang or Neroli as your water-based carrier. Choose 2-3 oils to add to your blend. You can use the chart to determine which essential oils you would like to add to your blend.

What You Will Need:

18 - 24 drops top note essential oil
12 - 16 drops middle essential oil
6 - 8 drops base essential oil
2 oz (60 ml) PET plastic or glass spray bottle
1/2 teaspoon Solubol or aloe vera gel
glass bowl and stir rod
funnel
perfume strips
2 oz hydrosol, floral water, or distilled water

What to Do:

1. Remove the spray nozzle from the spray bottle—you will add your carrier and oils right into the spray bottle.
2. Choose three essential oils. Add the number of drops for each note. Check the scent when adding drops to make sure you are happy with the scent.
3. Replace the nozzle and cap and shake.
4. Create a nice label for your room spray.

> A GENERAL RULE OF THUMB IN AROMATHERAPY IS THAT FOR EVERY YEAR YOU HAVE SUFFERED FROM A CHRONIC CONDITION, IT COULD TAKE ONE MONTH OF THERAPY TO CORRECT THE CONDITION.

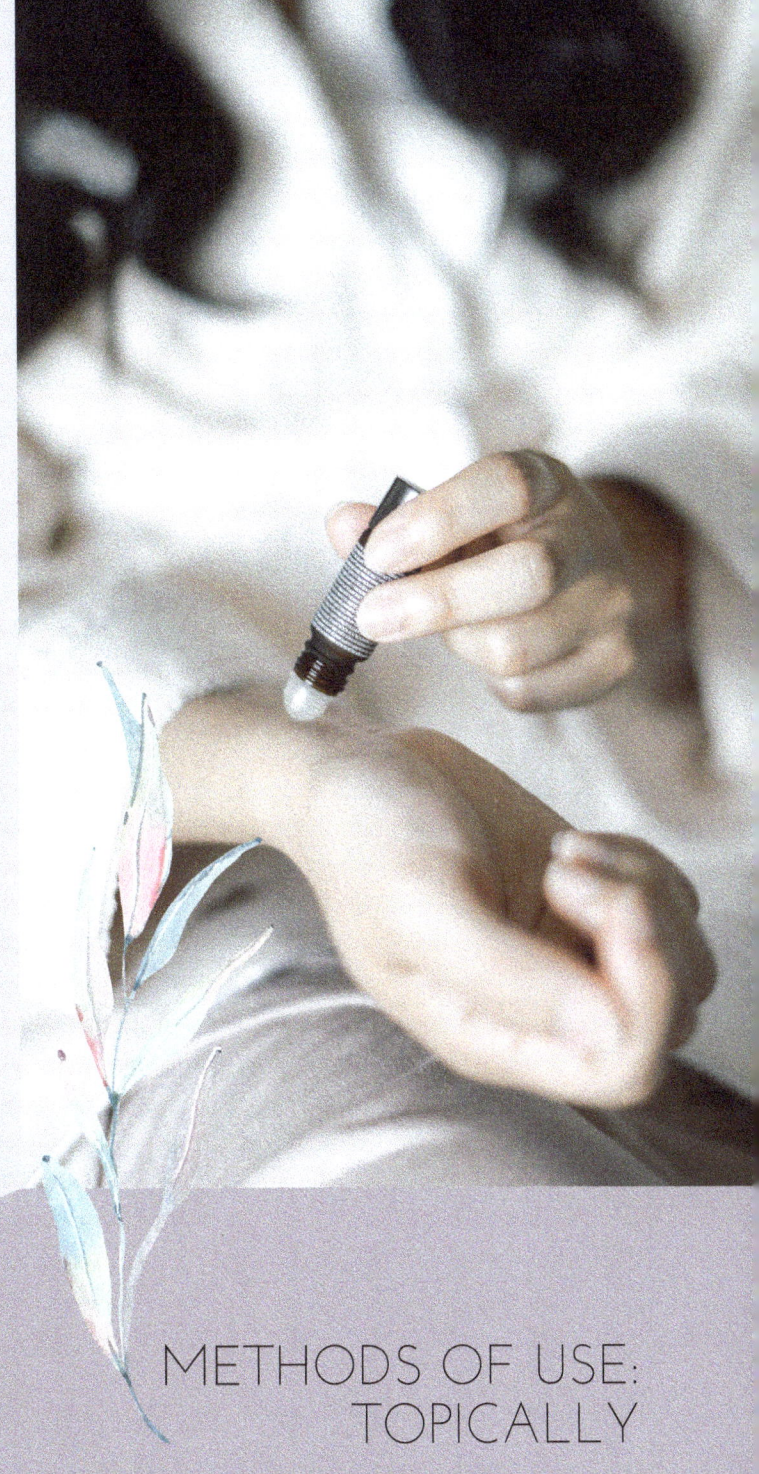

CHAPTER 9 —

METHODS OF USE: TOPICALLY

Topical use is applying the essential oils directly to the skin's surface; always use a carrier for topical use. Ways to use essential oils topically include:

- Roller Bottle
- Lotion
- Massage Oil
- Bath Salts

You can apply the essential oil(s) of choice to the back of the neck, feet, legs, etc., mixed with a lotion or carrier oil. Try combining a couple of oils to create a synergistic blend for multiple health benefits.

When using an essential oil topically, dilute it with a carrier oil. Essential oils are potent and direct application, or "neat," may cause irritation to the skin. Also, combining essential oils with a carrier base oil such as almond or coconut oil can add additional benefits to your treatment.

Topical application is one of the easiest and most effective ways to use essential oils. For example, massage stimulates blood circulation while reducing muscular tension, aches and pain, and inflammation. Also, it significantly reduces stress and can offer comfort and peace of mind, allowing you to sleep. Caution should be exercised when using topical aromatherapy preparations around drug injection sites or areas of the body where transdermal medications are in use (i.e., estrogen or nicotine patches, etc.).

The absorption of certain essential oil chemical compounds has been confirmed through analysis of blood concentrations, with maximum levels attained in as little as 10 minutes.

WAYS TO USE ESSENTIAL OILS TOPICALLY

Roll-On – Use a rollerball applicator to apply the oil blend where needed. Reapply several times a day as needed.

Rub On – Rub 1-2 drops of essential oil directly "neat" on the joint or affected area. Or rub an essential oil or essential oil blend on the bottom of your feet each evening before bed.

Massage – Massage an essential oil blend (with a carrier oil) over the body for several minutes. Reapply as desired. Apply to the back of the neck, joints, and feet. Applying essential oils topically can be quite beneficial since the oils will permeate your skin due to their transdermal properties. They stimulate circulation, help eliminate toxins, and absorb the minerals needed to function correctly. A variety of techniques used in massage therapy can incorporate the use of essential oils. Add 6-9 drops of essential oil to a tablespoon of your favorite carrier oil and massage into the body.

Bath – Sea salt baths are great for relaxation because they stimulate circulation. Sea salts and Epsom salts are great to use in baths. For a full bath, mix 8-10 drops of essential oil into two ounces of sea salts or a cup of milk, then pour into a running bath. Agitate water in a figure-eight motion to make sure the oil is mixed well, preventing irritation to mucous membranes. Another method is to add essential oils after the bath has been drawn. Mix essential oils into a palm full of liquid soap, shampoo, or a tablespoon of Jojoba oil and swish around to dissolve in the tub. Soak for 15-20 minutes.

Shower – While showering, add a drop or two of essential oil to a washcloth with liquid soap or body wash and rub it on the body.

Lotions/Cream – Blending essential oils in an unscented, natural lotion/cream base allow you to benefit from the therapeutic qualities of the essential oil, giving you a non-oily way to apply essential oils. This is especially useful for someone with a skin condition that does not do well with oils. The dilution rate for using essential oils in a lotion base is no more than 2%. For adults, use 20 drops of essential oil to four ounces of lotion. For children and the elderly, use ten drops of essential oil to four ounces of lotion.

Body Oil – Mix 30 drops of essential oil per ounce of cold-pressed carrier oil such as coconut oil. Choose an all-purpose oil that relieves stress, tension, and headaches and smells terrific.

MASSAGE OIL

Essential oils have been used for many years to enhance relaxation during a massage. Using an essential oil with a calming, relaxing property as part of a relaxing massage is a great way to promote positive feelings.

To apply, warm a few drops of essential oil with a teaspoon of a favorite carrier oil in your hand, rub between the palms, and then massage the oil into the temples or neck muscles. Massaging these two areas with essential oils is an effective way to calm and relax you.

This can also be applied to the shoulders, arms, back, legs, or feet to help relax these areas. Diluting essential oils with carrier oil will help absorb the oils into the skin and encourage relaxation. Please make sure the essential oil you choose is safe, as some are potent and could irritate the skin.

As a general rule of thumb: Use two to three drops of essential oil per teaspoon of carrier oil (follow individual recipes when available). A full-body massage takes approximately one ounce of carrier oil. Any natural carrier oil is okay to use when preparing a massage blend. As a general rule, add 10-12 drops of essential oil to 30ml carrier oil. For children and the elderly, use only 5-6 drops of essential oil to 30ml of carrier oil.

WHEN CHOOSING YOUR CARRIER OIL

Odor: A few carrier oils have a distinct odor. When added to an essential oil, it may alter the aroma.

Absorption: Your skin can absorb some carrier oils better than others.

Skin Type: Depending on your skin type, some oils may irritate or worsen a skin condition, such as acne.

Shelf Life: Some carrier oils can be stored longer than others without going bad.

> TOPICALLY IS ONE OF THE EASIEST AND MOST EFFECTIVE WAYS TO USE ESSENTIAL OILS.

CHAPTER 10 —

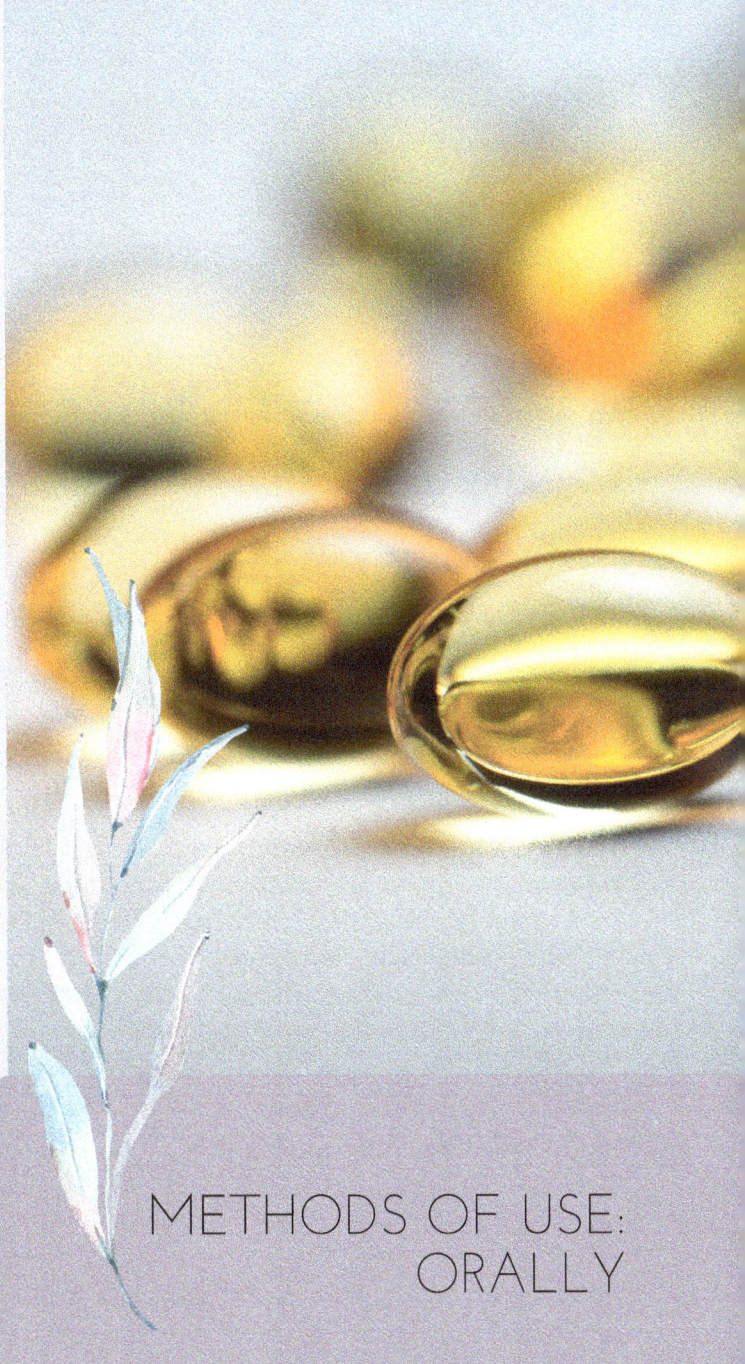

METHODS OF USE: ORALLY

Certain essential oils can be taken internally for relaxation. Check labels carefully to ensure the essential oils you choose are safe for ingestion. Not all essential oils are safe for taking orally.

If you are considering ingesting essential oils, you will want to treat your essential oils like powerful medicines because that is what they are. Taking an oil orally is nearly ten times stronger than when applied topically, so starting with a tiny amount and increasing gradually is wise. While many essential oils are safe when used internally, some are not. Be sure to read about the oil and do your research to know any warnings or contradictions. Also, you will want to be aware of proper dosage protocols. The necessary internal dose and frequency depend on age, size, and health condition, varying from person to person.

One essential oil company stated on its website, "The recommended internal dose of essential oils is 1-5 drops, depending on the oil or blend." Taking more than that is not advantageous; in fact, it can be harmful. It is better to take a smaller dose, which can be repeated every 4-6 hours as needed. A low daily dose is recommended for extended internal use.

Ingestion of certain essential oils may not be the most efficient method for absorption into the bloodstream. They are absorbed into systemic circulation via the digestive tract. However, essential oils may lose some active principal compounds when taken orally due to the first pass of hepatic metabolism.

There are several methods for taking essential oils. In this book, internal use will comprise consuming essential oils by mouth in a vegetable capsule, adding oil to honey, or on a sugar cube. Essential oils taken by mouth, not in a capsule, may be absorbed through the cheeks, tongue, or throat lining. Essential oils are highly concentrated and potent—treat like you would with any other highly concentrated pharmaceutical. When using essential oils internally, it is recommended to seek the advice of a certified medical practitioner who is also trained in aromatherapy or a

Clinical Certified Aromatherapist who is also trained in internal ingestion for the best protocol.

When using essential oils internally, doses in the range of one to three drops, one to two times a day (for adults), following a protocol appropriate for your health. Caution should be used as all essential oils are not recommended for ingestion. You should receive guidance from a qualified health professional before ingesting essential oils. Please store your oils in a safe place away from children. Using the appropriate amount of essential oil in a vegetable capsule that has been adequately diluted can be maximally absorbed by the gut for the whole-body effect. But like medicines, essential oil ingestion carries the potential for side effects, mild to severe, including seizures and poisoning.

Capsules – Gel capsules with fractionated coconut or olive oil are an optimum way to ingest harsh essential oils such as Cinnamon or Thyme. Such oils can be used for certain nervous system imbalances such as stress, insomnia, and anxiety. Add one or two drops of essential oil to a "00" gelatin capsule filled with a carrier oil such as olive or fractionated coconut oil to buffer the essential oil. Take orally as you would with traditional supplements. A single oil or essential oil blend may be used in this way. For example, a capsule is filled with 20% essential oil diluted with 80% vegetable oil (one ml=20 drops approximately). Each "00" capsule holds approximately 0.7-.91mL or 14 drops, and "0" capsules hold ten drops of oil. Enteric-Coated Gelatin Capsules could also be used since they do not release the essential oil until they are in the small intestine.

Juice or Water – Add one or two drops of essential oil to a small glass of juice. Stir to blend well, as oil will tend to float on the surface. Solubol can be added as a dispersant to distribute the oils.

Tea – Add one or two drops of essential oil to a teaspoon of honey and stir into a cup of tea or warm water. Be sure not to overheat the water, as oils will evaporate. Sip slowly.

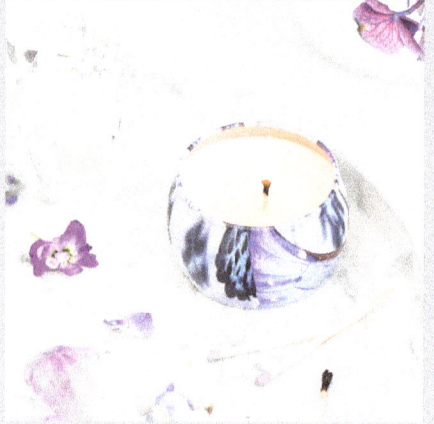

Swishing – Add several drops of essential oil to a cup of water and swish around the mouth before swallowing.

Sugar Cube – Use a dropper to add one or two drops of essential oil to a cube of sugar. It can be taken directly or added to a drink.

Honey – Essential oils can be blended with honey water. Mix 1-2 drops of essential oil into 1 tsp. honey, add warm water, and drink. Or add 1-2 drops of essential oil or oil blend to a tablespoon of honey, stir with a toothpick, and take orally.

RECOMMENDED DOSAGE

The recommended oral dosage with essential oils for adults is 1-3 drops, two to three times a day. The maximum daily dose is 12 drops. Some essential oil websites recommend up to 20 drops a day, which is relatively high and is therefore not recommended. Some professionals recommend using essential oils two weeks out of the month or taking one drop three times a day for an extended period. Others suggest using 1-2 drops twice daily for five days and taking two days' rest. Either way, taking breaks in your essential oil usage is advisable.

NEUTRAL TABLET

Neutral tablets are another widely used excipient for essential oils. They dissolve quickly and are absorbed in the mucosa of the mouth. For safety, ensure the tablet has completely absorbed the essential oils before swallowing it. You can swallow the tablet once it has dried.

Other alternatives include sugar cubes, bread, charcoal, rice flour capsules, syrups, and dried powdered herb capsules.

MIXING ESSENTIAL OILS IN WATER

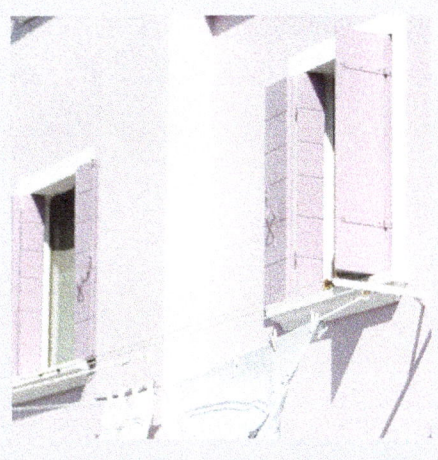

To emulsify the essential oils in the water, two products help make them more soluble: Solubol and Dispera. These are recommended to reduce throat irritation and digestive issues.

Solubol is a natural, non-alcoholic dispersant that quickly disperses essential oils into the water. Blend one part of essential oil with four parts of Solubol. Shake well. Add 3-4 drops to a glass of water or juice. This is also an excellent way to use essential oils in the bath.

Dispera is similar to Solubol but contains a 70% alcohol solution. Dispera also aids the absorption of essential oils by the digestive tract. Combine 80-90% Dispera with 20-10% essential oil and place one to two drops in a glass of water.

WHY TAKE ESSENTIAL OILS BY MOUTH?

It is widely believed that essential oils are suitable for anxiety, sleeplessness, and other related conditions. Essential oils safe for internal use can be absorbed through the mucous membranes (nose, under the tongue, and the throat lining). The oral route ushers essential oils into the digestive tract, readily absorbing them into the bloodstream. Some of the issues that respond to this method include:
- Relaxation
- Insomnia
- Anxiety

WHEN SHOULD YOU TAKE ESSENTIAL OILS INTERNALLY?

Essential oils should typically be taken before a meal. Another option, especially when taking strong combinations (like Thyme and Cinnamon), is to take it halfway through a meal to not upset or irritate the stomach lining.

THE SUBLINGUAL ROUTE

The word 'sublingual' refers to applications placed under the tongue. Essential oils are administered by placing one drop of essential oil under the tongue or by placing one or two drops on a neutral tablet and placing the tablet under the tongue to dissolve.

This method speeds the absorption of the molecules into the bloodstream and avoids the effect of hepatic first-pass metabolism and the gastrointestinal tract. It is most readily absorbed in this manner.

The reticulated vein underneath the tongue absorbs the essential oil components. It then transports them from the tiny facial veins to the larger jugular and brachiocephalic veins.

Advantages of Sublingual Dosing:

- Fast-acting (peak levels reached in 10-15 minutes)
- Easy to self-administer
- Bypasses extensive hepatic first-pass metabolic process
- Sublingual dosing does not require swallowing, which is suitable for patients with Dysphagia
- The absorption rate is 3 to 10 times greater than through the oral route

WHEN TO USE THE SUBLINGUAL ROUTE AND DOSAGE?

The sublingual route is recommended for acute insomnia or acute anxiety.

DOSAGE

Sublingual dosage: 6 drops of essential per day maximum for adults with 1 to 3 drops per dose of non-irritating essential oils.

For adults: 1-2 drops three-four times per day
For adolescents: 2 drops two times per day
For children over seven years old: 1 drop two times per day

When taking sublingual drops, it is recommended to use an eye dropper and bring it in front of a mirror to be sure the application gets under the tongue. You may also use it on a neutral tablet as well.

Buccal dosage: for mouth conditions, place one drop of essential oil in the mouth between the upper and lower gums and cheek area. This can also be placed on neutral tablets.

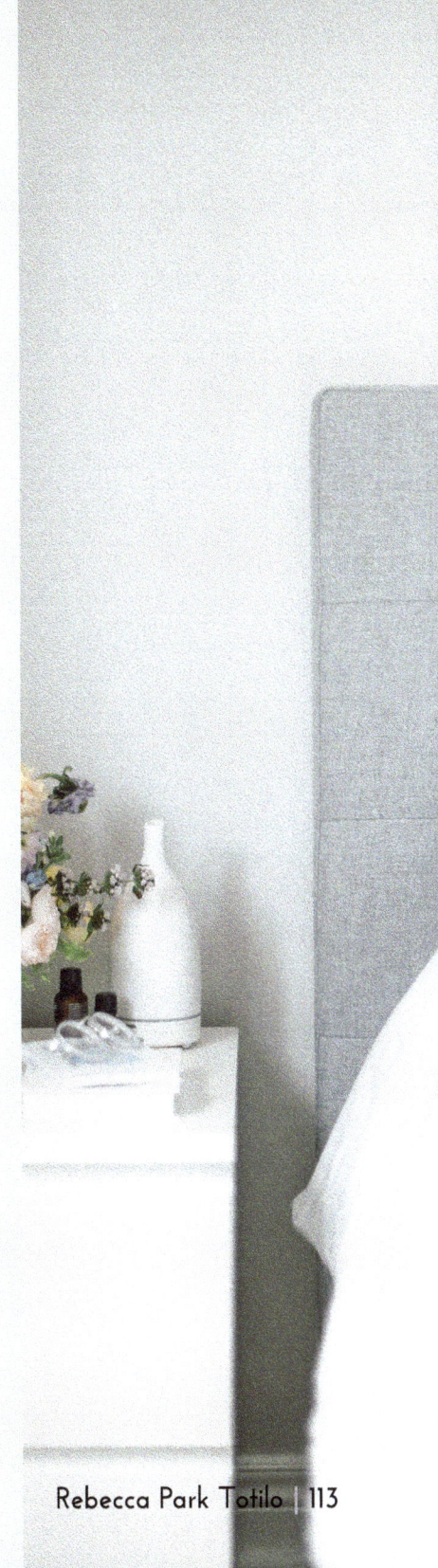

When to use: The best time to take sublingual essential oils is before eating a meal.

WHICH ESSENTIAL OILS SHOULD YOU USE FOR SUBLINGUAL USE?

You should use only non-irritating essential oils such as Lavender, Coriander Seed, Lemon, etc. The only downside to this is possibly an unpleasant taste based on the flavor of the oils.

HOW LONG SHOULD I USE ESSENTIAL OILS?

It is recommended to continue essential oil therapy for a few days or more following relief of symptoms to ensure complete healing occurs. A general rule of thumb in aromatherapy is that for every year you have suffered from a chronic condition, it could take one month of therapy to correct the condition. For acute conditions, if you do not obtain results within an hour or so, try a different essential oil or method of application. Everyone responds differently, and you may need to use more or less essential oil, depending on how your body reacts.

BUILDING UP A TOLERANCE TO ESSENTIAL OILS

It is safe to use the recipes in this book, as recommended, several times a day for a week or more. It is recommended to limit the use of the same oil or essential oil blend to twenty-one days and then take a week's break. Rotating your blends and using different oils or blends are also recommended.

ROTATE YOUR OILS

After regularly using the same oil or blend, you should rotate your blends and use different oils. This is recommended for two reasons. First, this reduces the possibility of a risk of sensitization to the essential oil or blend that you are using.

Secondly, this also reduces the chance of your body developing resistance or becoming acclimated to the effectiveness of the essential oils you are using. In other words, the essential oil blend may no longer work or provide the same positive benefits it once did.

ESSENTIAL OIL SAFETY

In general, essential oils are safe for aromatherapy and therapeutic purposes. Nevertheless, safety must be exercised due to their potency and high concentration. Please read and follow these guidelines to obtain the maximum effectiveness and benefits.

- Avoid sunbathing, tanning booths, or saunas immediately after applying essential oils topically.
- Be careful to avoid getting essential oils in the eyes. If you splash a drop or two of essential oil in the eyes, use a small amount of olive oil (or another carrier oil) to dilute the essential oil and absorb it with a washcloth. If severe, seek medical attention immediately.
- Take extra precautions when using oils with children. Never use undiluted essential oils on babies, and always store your essential oils out of the reach of children.
- If a dangerous quantity of essential oil has been ingested, immediately drink olive oil and induce vomiting. The olive oil will help slow down its absorption and dilute the essential oil. Do not drink water—this will speed up the essential oil absorption.
- Never use oils undiluted on your skin. Always dilute with a carrier oil. Stop using oil immediately if there is redness, burning, itching, or irritation. Be sure to wash your hands after handling pure, undiluted essential oils.
- If you are pregnant, lactating, suffer from epilepsy, have cancer, liver damage, or another medical condition, use essential oils under the care and supervision of a qualified Aromatherapist or medical practitioner.
- Less is best when taking essential oils internally. Take fewer drops every 4-6 hours versus more at one time.

CHAPTER 11

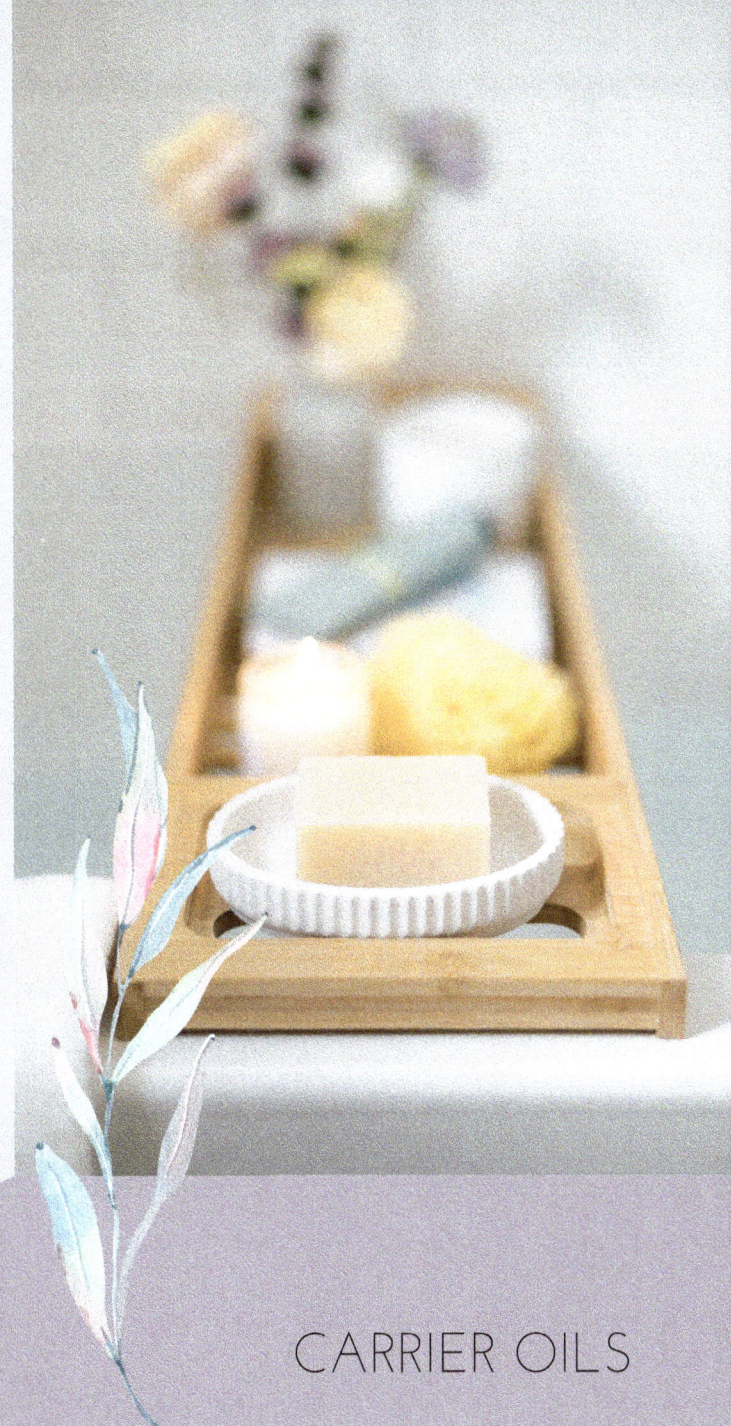

CARRIER OILS

When you use essential oils topically, you will want to dilute them with a carrier or vegetable oil. Carrier and infused oils are used to dilute essential oils and absolutes by offering the necessary lubrication and moisture to the skin for aromatherapy.

Carrier oils come from nuts, seeds, or kernels that contain essential fatty acids, fat-soluble vitamins, minerals, and other crucial nutrients. You will find a variety of carrier oils to choose from, each possessing different therapeutic properties.

Distinct from essential oils, carrier oils do not contain aromatic scents (or only a very faint scent) and evaporate due to their large molecular structure. For this reason, most consider carrier oils just a vehicle for applying essential oils to the skin in massage. However, they offer healing properties that essential oils do not possess. Your aromatherapy experience can be significantly enhanced by choosing the best combination of carrier and essential oils.

SHELF LIFE OF CARRIER OILS

A carrier oil's shelf life, the length of time before a particular oil begins to turn rancid, can be significantly influenced by heat and light. You will want to store your oils in a cool, dark place to preserve their freshness and, in some cases, refrigerate, as heat and sunlight can shorten their shelf life. When refrigerating, oils may appear cloudy but will regain their transparency upon returning to room temperature. If you have a large amount of carrier oil on hand, you can freeze the unused portion until ready for use.

Carrier Oil	Shelf Life
Almond (sweet)	12 months
Apricot Kernel	6-12 months
Argan	24 months
Avocado	12 months
Borage	6 months
Carrot Seed	12 months
Cocoa Butter	3-5 years
Coconut (fractionated)	Indefinite
Coconut (virgin)	2-4 years
Evening Primrose	6-12 months
Grapeseed	3-6 months
Hemp Seed	12 months
Jojoba	Indefinite
Olive	12-18 months
Safflower	24 months
Shea Butter	Indefinite
Walnut	12 months

When carrier oils are used with essential oils topically, they provide a mechanism for the volatile oils to be transported more effectively. Most essential oils, when applied externally, move through the body system in an hour. A carrier oil, thicker than a volatile oil, "holds" the essential oil in place, delivering longer-lasting healing.

Essential oils in aromatherapy are highly concentrated and potent. Although there are only a few exceptions to using essential oils 'neat' or undiluted (such as Lavender and Chamomile), it is ideal always to use a carrier oil with your essential oils to avoid having an adverse effect or skin irritation.

TIP: A massage oil blend with 10-15% essential oil and 85-90% carrier oil will ensure a powerful massage oil that is smooth and great-smelling.

Carrier oils provide the much-needed lubrication, allowing hands to move freely over the skin, and helping absorb essential oils into the body. Choose a carrier oil that is light, non-sticky, and can effectively penetrate the skin. Always check the label to ensure it's 100% pure, unrefined, and cold-pressed.

Tip: Try not to mix too much of your favorite massage blend in advance if you don't plan on using it right away.

With the vast selection of carrier oils, each with various therapeutic benefits, choosing one will depend on the area it's being applied to, the treatment plan, and any skin sensitivities. When using oil for massage, viscosity is an important consideration. Some carrier oils may work better than others in specific applications. For example, Grapeseed oil is generally very thin, while Olive oil is much thicker, and others, such as Sunflower and Sweet Almond, have viscosities halfway between these extremes. You can easily blend carrier oils to combine their properties of viscosity, absorption rate, and benefits.

Almond Oil

Almond Oil is one of the most useful, practical, and moderately priced carrier oils. It is ideal for all skin types as it moisturizes and reconditions the skin with its satiny smooth texture. This pale-yellow oil quickly absorbs into the skin, leaving your skin feeling soft and non-greasy. Sweet Almond relieves itching, soreness, dryness, and inflammation and is especially beneficial for eczema. As a lightly nutty refined oil rich in fatty acids, proteins, and vitamin D, it is everyone's favorite massage base oil for loosening stiff muscles and achy joints.

Dilution: Can be used at 100%.

Coconut Oil (Fractionated)

Coconut Oil (Fractionated) seems to be quickly becoming the carrier oil of choice because of its broad use in alternative medicine and healing. While it is fractionated, no change has been made chemically. Instead, its molecular structure 'fraction' has been separated, allowing it to remain liquid at room temperature, making it much more helpful in aromatherapy. Coconut oil is perfect as a moisturizer for the body while delivering its many health benefits. Its light, easily absorbable texture gives skin a smooth satin effect with virtually no scent of its own and indefinite shelf life.

Dilution: Can be used at 100%.

Coconut Oil (Virgin)

Coconut Oil (Virgin) has an incredible balance of natural saturated fatty acids with antibacterial and antiviral properties not found in other oils. Coconut oil is perfect as a skin conditioner for nearly all skin conditions and is believed to stimulate hair growth. It has a light, aromatic coconut scent that becomes solid at room temperature. For this reason, blending with other carrier oils in your body care products is recommended. It is fully digestible and is considered a healthy cooking oil. Several virgin coconut oils are high in antioxidants which are positively associated with reducing oxidative stress and thus lowering blood pressure.

Dilution: It can be used alone directly, but it is recommended to use 10-25% dilution with other carrier oils.

Grapeseed Oil

Grapeseed Oil is a lovely, light green, and odorless oil, useful as a base oil for many creams, lotions, and carrier oil. Grapeseed oil is pressed from the seeds of a grape and contains OPCs, flavonoids, vitamin E, resveratrol, and fatty acids. It is non-allergenic and has very high levels of linoleic acid, with traces of proanthocyanidins, which are very potent antioxidants. It is especially beneficial for all skin types because of its natural non-allergenic properties. Grapeseed works well, especially when other oils do not absorb well, without leaving a greasy feeling after application. Grapeseed makes an ideal carrier oil for body massage bases. Saturation takes longer than some other carrier oils.

Dilution: Can be used at 100%.

Jojoba Oil

Jojoba Oil is bright and golden in color and is known as one of the best oils (actually a liquid wax) for hair and skin. It penetrates the skin quickly and is excellent for nourishing and healing inflamed skin, psoriasis, eczema, or dermatitis. It is suitable for all skin types and promotes a healthy, glowing complexion by gently unclogging the pores and lifting embedded impurities. Jojoba is suitable for all aromatherapy uses other than a full-body massage. And, because of the oil's antioxidants, it does not become rancid and can even prevent rancidity in other oils.

Dilution: It can be used at 100%, but many use a 10% dilution with other carrier oils due to its price.

Olive Oil (Extra Virgin)

Olive Oil (Extra Virgin) is light to medium green in color with a slightly dense texture. It is very soothing and carries disinfecting and healing properties. Olive oil is legendary since it has been used over the centuries for multiple purposes, but due to its overpowering scent, this oil does not work well for massages. However, it is beneficial in some lotions for burns or scars. Olive is very helpful for dry, damaged, or split hair and is soothing for inflamed skin such as eczema. The "virgin" indicates it comes from the first pressing of the fruit. The "extra" means it comes from a single source. Extra virgin olive oil is beneficial for high blood pressure because it contains more vitamin E than virgin, pure or extra light varieties.

Dilution: Can be used at 100% or 25-50% dilution with another carrier oil blend.

Shea Butter

Shea Butter is a thick, lustrous butter (not a carrier oil) with excellent therapeutic properties. It contains powerful anti-inflammatory properties known to reduce swelling and pain. Shea butter leaves the skin feeling smooth and healthy and combats many skin conditions. Shea butter has a very cream-like consistency, so you may want to warm it and blend it with other carrier oils for a thinner or liquid consistency if desired.

Dilution: Can be used at 100% or diluted at 25-25% with another carrier oil for blending purposes.

TIP: Mineral oil and petroleum jelly should never be used as a carrier oil in therapeutic blending. These are derivatives of petroleum products from gasoline and are not of natural botanical origins. It prevents toxins from escaping the body through perspiration and is believed to also prevent the body from adequately absorbing vitamins and utilizing them, including essential oil absorption.

DILUTION RATE FOR YOUR BLENDS

When creating an essential oil blend for sleep, you will need to consider the amount of carrier oil to use for dilution. Be sure to dilute correctly to make sure your blend is safe to use and doesn't waste your precious essential oil.

The following dilution rate chart shows you the amount of pure therapeutic essential oil to use with your carrier oil. Use a measuring spoon to add the carrier oil and a dropper to add your essential oils.

Most essential oils should be diluted for topical applications, using a 1-3% concentration of essential oils (in some cases, 5-10%). This means 6-24 drops of essential oil will be used per ounce of carrier. Therapeutic massage blends will contain between 1-5% essential oils.

For example, adding two to three drops of pure essential oil will need diluting by adding about a teaspoon of carrier oil. For children or senior citizens, cut this amount in half.

SIMPLE EVERYDAY DILUTION CHART

Essential Oil	To	Carrier Oil
1 drop		¼ teaspoon
2-5 drops		1 teaspoon
4-10 drops		2 teaspoons
6-15 drops		1 Tablespoon
8-20 drops		4 teaspoons
12-30 drops		2 Tablespoons

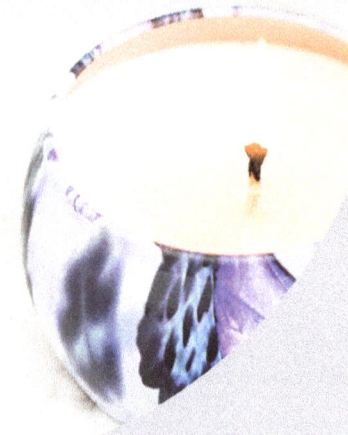

EQUIPMENT USED FOR CREATING BLENDS FOR EMOTIONS

Before getting started, you will want to gather your supplies, such as bottles, droppers, and containers. Below is a list of the necessary tools you will need to have on hand:

Glass Bottles, preferably dark, in 5ml, 10ml, and 15ml sizes with orifice reducers (plastic dropper), can be used to make topical essential oil blends.

Glass Spray Bottles are great for making room sprays, facial spritzers, or cleaning solutions. You will find these in sizes 1-ounce, 2-ounce, 4-ounce, 8-ounce, and 16-ounce.

Small Glass Tubs are perfect for bath salts, facial creams, salves, scrubs, or other bath blends. These come in various shapes and sizes, from 2-ounce to 8-ounce.

Pocket Diffusers are perfect as "personal inhalers" to carry in a pocket or purse with your favorite blend. They come with a cotton wick that saturates the essential oil inside the chamber. These are terrific for taking to work or school!

Waterproof Labels will prevent ink from running. Be sure to name each product and add the date you made the product. You will need waterproof labels in all shapes and sizes.

MAKING YOUR FIRST EMOTION BLEND

Now that you have learned how many drops of each note to use in your essential oil blend and have checked the precautions, it's time to start blending.

1. Gather all the necessary equipment: bottles, pipettes, essential oils, paper towels, labels, vials, and containers.

2. Ensure the counter space is clean and the area you work in is well-ventilated. You may want to put down wax paper (or a paper towel) to prevent any damage to the countertop from accidental spills. This will also make cleaning up much more manageable.

3. If you are using essential oils that are new to you, place one drop of the oil on a test strip (or small piece of paper) and wave it under your nose. Inhale the fragrance. If this fragrance is not what you had in mind, choose another oil and test it again. You will want to do this with each oil until you have settled on the ones you want to use for your blend. It is a good idea to have a can of coffee grounds to smell after each fragrance to clear your palette.

4. Once you have chosen the three oils for your blend, wave all three test strips fanned out beneath your nose and see if you like them. Remember that if you despise the scent, you may hesitate to use it regularly.

5. Check the safety precautions for the essential oils you have chosen to ensure there aren't any contradictions. Always consider any other health conditions, such as epilepsy or medications, that may cause an adverse effect. Safety precautions must always be considered for the method you choose in their usage and for the person you are formulating the blend for.

6. Choose a new, clean bottle to use. Using a pipette, extract each essential oil into the bulb to place in your bottle. You may need to squeeze more than once to get the desired amount. Remember to use a separate pipette or glass eye dropper for each oil used. Add your base note essential oil first, one drop at a time. This is typically the most viscous or thickest oil. Next, add the middle note essential oil, followed by the top note essential oil. Use only the exact number of drops your recipe calls for. One drop of too many can alter the results. Replace the cap on the bottle and shake to mix oils.

7. Add your essential oil blend to a carrier oil (lotion, gel, sea salts, etc.) and blend well to distribute the oils. What you use as your carrier and how much to add will depend on which application method (Massage Blend, Bath Blend, Room Spray, etc.) you choose.

TIP: Always leave ½ inch of headspace at the top of your bottle allowing your pure essential oil blend to breathe and expand.

CHAPTER 12

RECIPES

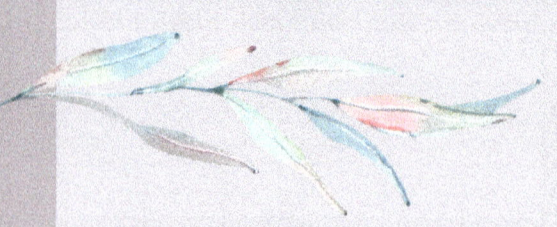

BASIC MASSAGE OIL BLEND

Here is an easy-to-follow basic recipe for making a massage blend! You get to decide which essential oils to use depending on the type of massage and the effect you are looking to achieve.

What You Will Need:

1-ounce (30 ml) Carrier Oil, Lotion, or Gel
9-15 drops Top Note essential oil
6-10 drops Middle Note essential oil
3-5 drops Base Note essential oil
Glass Bottle

What To Do:

1. Pour your carrier oil, lotion, or gel into a clean bottle.
2. Add your essential oils one drop at a time, starting with your base note, the middle note, and then the top note.
3. Shake well to mix oils and carrier.
4. Add a label with the name, ingredients, and date created.
5. Use it two to three times a day.

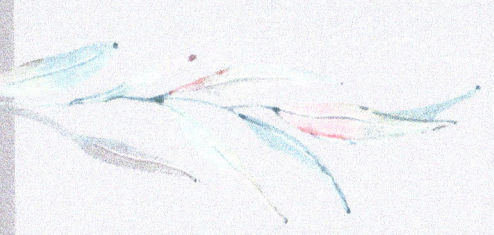

BASIC BATH SALTS BLEND

You can use Dead Sea, Himalayan, or Epsom salts for this basic bath salts recipe. Soak in a bath with this incredible blend to soothe the day's stress. Your bath salts can be made in advance and stored in a pretty container for convenience.

What You Will Need:

2 cups Epsom Salts
1 cup Sea Salts
1 cup Baking Soda
30 drops Top Note essential oil
20 drops Middle Note essential oil
10 drops Base Note essential oil
Wide Mouth Jar or Container

What To Do:

1. Add essential oils together in a container. Stir to mix.
2. Add sea salts and mix well to saturate the salts with the oils thoroughly.
3. Add bath salts to a running bath and swish in the tub to mix thoroughly.

Tip: Check precautions for oils that may cause skin sensitivity. It is not recommended for children.

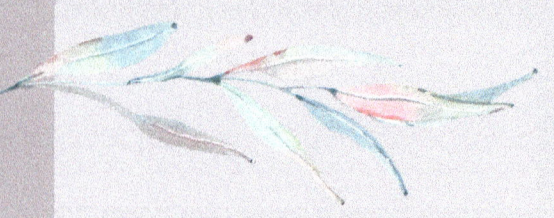

BASIC BATH OIL BLEND

After a long day, soaking in a warm bath with a relaxing essential oil blend can be a delightful treat. Not only does it help take the edge off tense muscles, but it also ensures a better night's sleep.

What You Will Need:

1 cup Almond Oil or Coconut oil
30 drops Top Note essential oil
20 drops Middle Note essential oil
10 drops Base Note essential oil
Corked container
Crystal beads, dried flowers, tiny seashells, etc. (Optional)

What To Do:

1. Pour the carrier oil through a funnel into the corked container, leaving about an inch at the top.
2. Add essential oils to the container. Stir well to mix.
3. Cork the container and agitate the bottle gently.
4. Let it sit for 2-3 days before use. Add decor to your bottle.
5. For use, pour ½-1 teaspoon into the palm of your hand and gently massage into the body after a bath.

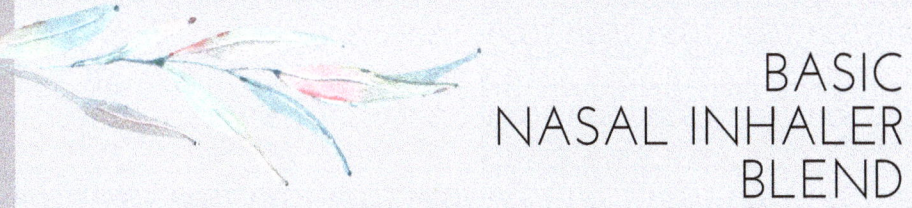

BASIC NASAL INHALER BLEND

Filling a new nasal inhaler with your essential oil blend is an effective way to experience the therapeutic power of essential oils. Inhalers are also great to use for many emotions, including anxiety and restlessness. They are small enough to carry in a pocket or purse and have on hand for immediate relief. Add 15-18 drops of your essential oil blend to your inhaler.

What You Will Need:

9 drops Top Note essential oil
6 drops Middle Note essential oil
3 drops Base Note essential oil
Glass Dropper
Small Plastic Inhaler

What To Do:

1. In a container, mix essential oils. Stir well to mix.
2. Use a glass or disposal dropper to fill the nasal inhaler.
3. Carry and take a whiff as needed.

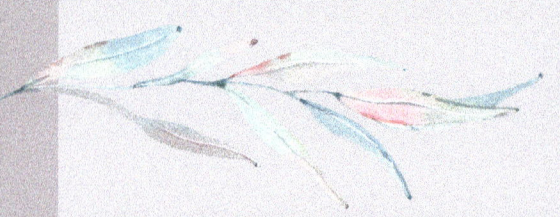

BASIC FOOT OIL BLEND

A luxurious foot treatment with essential oils can readily deliver healing throughout the body. The sensitive skin and tissues of the feet take a lot of abuse and deserve a special blend that can easily be massaged in.

What You Will Need:

1 ounce (30ml) Almond oil
3 drops Top Note essential oil
2 drops Middle Note essential oil
1 drop Base Note essential oil
1-ounce Glass Bottle

What To Do:

1. In a container, mix essential oils. Stir well to combine.
2. Add carrier oil to the bottle, replace the lid and shake to blend.
3. Massage oil blend into feet after a bath or shower or before bed. Wear soft, cotton socks to bed.

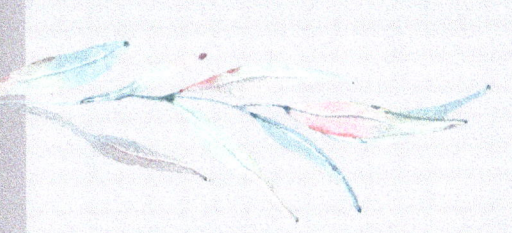

BASIC CAPSULE BLEND

Here is a simple recipe for making an essential oil capsule. It is one of the best ways to take essential oils internally and bypass unpleasant tastes. You can use 1-2 drops of essential oil per capsule (depending on size).

What You Will Need:

1-2 drops Essential Oil* (20%)
Carrier Oil (80%)

What To Do:

1. Separate the two parts of the capsule. Remove the top half (wider cap). You will only be filling the bottom half.
2. Add essential oil directly into the capsule, one drop at a time, using a glass dropper. This needs to be done carefully; do not add too many drops or drip oil on the side of the capsule, which will make it sticky.
3. Fill the remaining space with olive, coconut, pomegranate oil, etc.
4. Take the capsule immediately after filling it. These capsules will begin to dissolve right after filling them.
5. Take one capsule once in the morning and once in the evening or as prescribed by your healthcare provider.

*Only use essential oils that are safe to ingest.

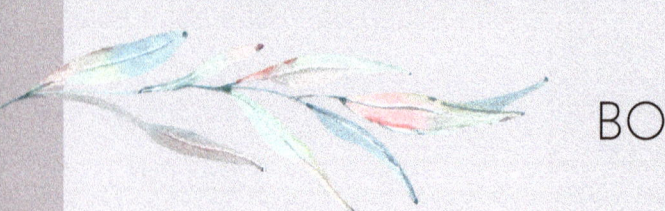

BASIC BODY LOTION BLEND

Do you want to try a good body lotion recipe? Why not make your own by following these simple instructions?

What You Will Need:

4 ounces Unscented Lotion, Hydrosol, or carrier oil
18 drops Top Note essential oil
12 drops Middle Note essential oil
6 drops Base Note essential oil
Glass Bottle or container

What To Do:

1. Add carrier oil to the container.
2. Add essential oils, starting with your base note essential oil first, then the middle note, and finally the top note essential oil.
3. Recap and shake well to mix.
4. Use it two to three times a day.

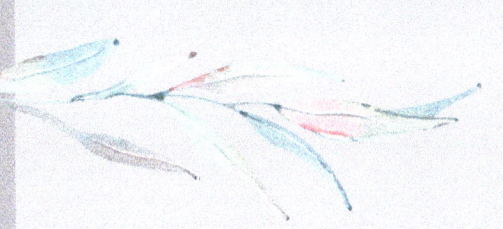

BASIC ROLL-ON BLEND

This basic recipe can be used to create a roll-on bottle applicator for your essential oil blend, depending on the oils you have on hand. Keep track of what you add or change, so you'll know how to make your favorite blends later.

What You Will Need:

½ ounce Jojoba oil
9 drops Top Note essential oil
6 drops Middle Note essential oil
3 drops Base Note essential oil
Glass Roller Bottle

What To Do:

1. Add your carrier oil, such as Jojoba, to a dark container.
2. When adding essential oils, start with the base note and then add the middle note, followed by the top note. As you add each one, check the scent to ensure it is what you want.
3. Insert the ball and apply it 2-3 times daily.

> WHEN SHOPPING FOR A GOOD QUALITY CARRIER OIL, MAKE SURE IT'S COLD-PRESSED TO RETAIN ALL OF ITS NATURAL QUALITIES.

CHAPTER 13

OTHER BOOKS BY REBECCA PARK TOTILO

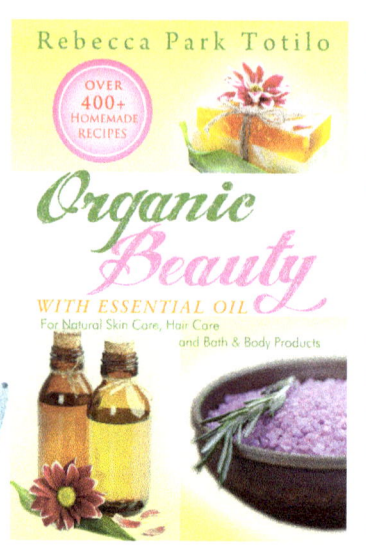

Organic Beauty With Essential Oil: Over 400+ Homemade Recipes for Natural Skin Care, Hair Care and Bath & Body Products

Sweep aside all those harmful chemically-based cosmetics and make your own organic bath and body products at home with the magic of potent essential oils! In this book, you'll find a luxurious array of over 400 eco-friendly recipes that call for breathtaking fragrances and soothing, rich organic ingredients satisfying you head to toe. Included you'll find helpful tips you can have the confidence knowing which essential oil to use and how much when creating your own body scrub, lip butter, or lotion bar! Discover how easy it is to make bath treats like fragrant shower gels, dreamy bubble baths, luscious creams and lotions, deep cleansing masks and facials for literally pennies using essential oils and ingredients from your kitchen.

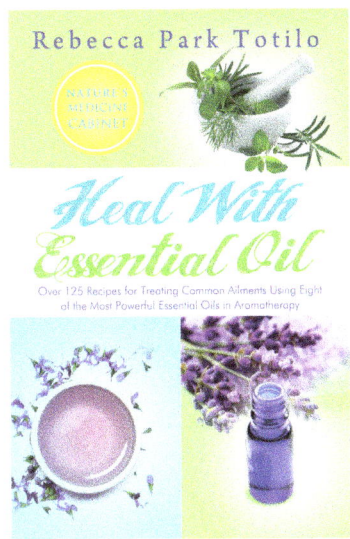

Heal With Essential Oil: Nature's Medicine Cabinet

Using essential oils drawn from nature's own medicine cabinet of flowers, trees, seeds and roots, man can tap into God's healing power to heal oneself from almost any pain. Find relief from many conditions and rejuvenate the body. With over 125 recipes, this practical guide will walk you through in the most easy-to-understand form how to treat common ailments with your essential oils for everyday living. Filled with practical advice on therapeutic blending of oils and safety, a directory of the most effective oils for common ailments and easy to follow remedies chart, and prescriptive blends for aches, pains and sicknesses.

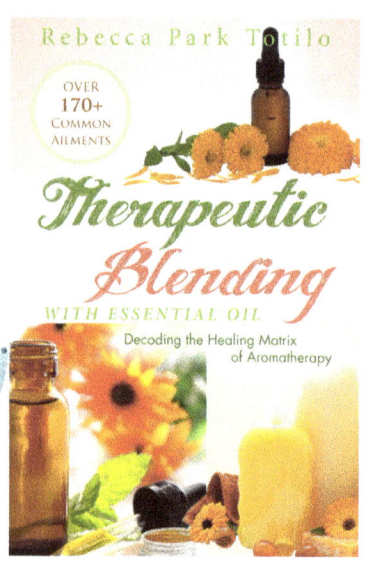

Therapeutic Blending With Essential Oil: Decoding the Healing Matrix of Aromatherapy

Therapeutic Blending With Essential Oil unlocks the healing power of essential oils and guides you through the intricate matrix of aromatherapy, with a compilation of over 170 common ailments. Discover how to properly formulate a blend for any physical or emotional symptom with easy to follow customizable recipes. Now, you can make your own massage oils, hand and body lotions, bath gels, compresses, salve ointments, smelling salts, nasal inhalers and more. This exhaustive guide takes all the guesswork out of blending oils from how many drops to include in a blend, to measuring thick oils, to how often to apply it for acute or chronic conditions. It also shows you how to create a single blend for multiple conditions. Even if you run out of oil for a favorite recipe, this book shows you how to substitute it with another oil.

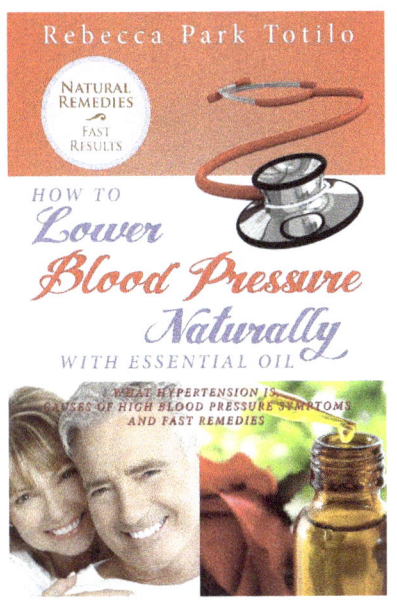

How To Lower Blood Pressure Naturally With Essential Oil: What Hypertension Is, Causes of High Pressure Symptoms and Fast Remedies

One out of three adults have it, and another one-third don't realize it. Oftentimes, it goes undetected for years. Even those who take multiple medications for it still don't have it under control. It's no secret—high blood pressure is rampant in America. High blood pressure, or hypertension, has become a household term. Between balancing meds and monitoring diets though, are the true causes—and best treatments—hidden in the shadows? In How to Lower Blood Pressure Naturally With Essential Oil, Rebecca Park Totilo sheds light on what high blood pressure is, the causes and symptoms of high blood pressure, and which essential oils regulate blood pressure and how to use essential oils as a natural, alternative method.

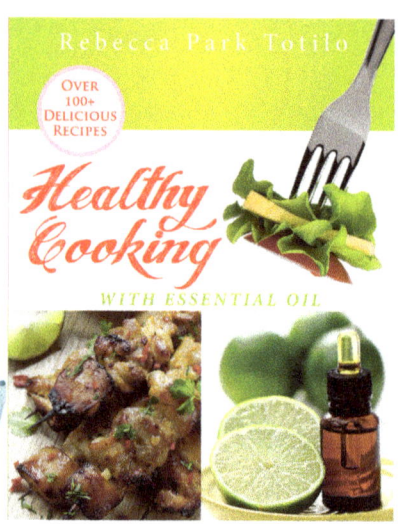

Healthy Cooking with Essential Oil

Imagine transforming an everyday dish into something extraordinary! Essential oils can enliven everything from soups, salads, to main dishes and desserts. Boasting flavor and fragrance, these intense essences can turn a dull, boring meal into something appetizing and delicious. Essential oils are fun, easy-to use and beneficial, compared to the traditional stale, dried herbs and spices found in most pantries today. Healthy food should never be thought of as mere fuel for the body, it should be enjoyed as a multi-sensory experience that brings therapeutic value as well as nourishment. For years we have limited the use of essential oils to scented candles and soaps, in the belief that they were unsafe to consume (and some are!). However, more people are realizing the value of using pure essential oils to enhance their diet. In Healthy Cooking With Essential Oil, you will learn how cooking with essential oils can open up a wealth of creative opportunities in the kitchen.

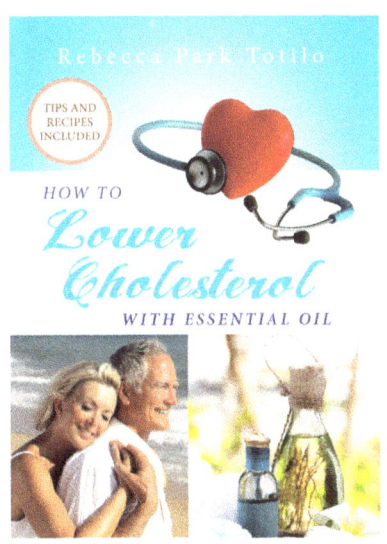

How to Lower Cholesterol with Essential Oil

Take healthy steps now to control high cholesterol and its risk factors with essential oils. People with high cholesterol have twice the risk for heart disease according to the Center for Disease Control and Prevention. What's worse, most folks aren't even aware that they have atherosclerosis until they have a heart attack or stroke. Lowering your cholesterol and triglycerides with essential oils may slow, reduce, or even stop the buildup of dangerous plaque in your arteries causing blockage of blood flow which could result in a heart attack or stroke. In this indispensable guide, author Rebecca Park Totilo presents scientific research supporting the efficacy of certain essential oils for lowering cholesterol, an extensive essential oil and carrier oil directory, natural treatments with recipes, along with easy-to-follow methods of use via inhalation, topically, and ingestion.

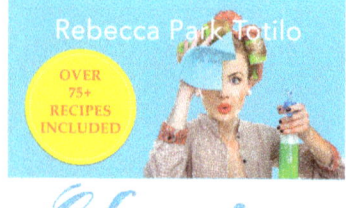
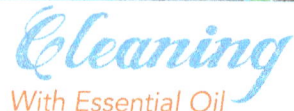
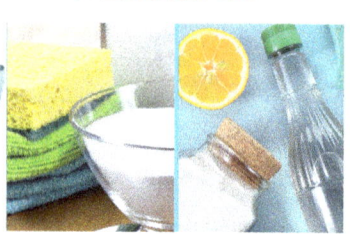

Cleaning With Essential Oil

Now you can have a clean, healthy home free from harsh chemicals using a few ingredients from your pantry and essential oils! Cleaning With Essential Oil features over 75 easy-to-make recipes for every household chore, including laundry detergent, heavy-duty oven cleaner, carpet deodorizer, antibacterial wipes, stain remover, and many more!

Essential oils expert Rebecca Park Totilo guides you in choosing the best essential oils for cleaning based on their chemistry, the health benefits of cleaning with essential oils, and tips for tackling the toughest cleaning jobs from cleaning kitchen appliances to disinfecting bathrooms. The best part is she shows you how to get the entire house clean in less than an hour! Complete shopping lists for supplies and essential oils are provided, so you have everything you need for making your homemade cleaners. Now, you can turn every room into a safe and toxic-free haven for family and pets to enjoy with products like

- Simple Citrus Soft Scrub
- Stainless Steel Appliance Spray
- Lavender Hand Foaming Soap
- Peppermint Daily Shower Spray
- Minty Fresh Window & Mirror Cleaner
- Garbage Disposal Cleaning Bombs
- Lemon and Geranium Swifty Floor Wipes

In Cleaning With Essential Oil, author Rebecca Park Totilo teaches you how to make your own "green cleaners" without spending a fortune while helping save the planet! Isn't it time you ditch the chemicals and make the switch?

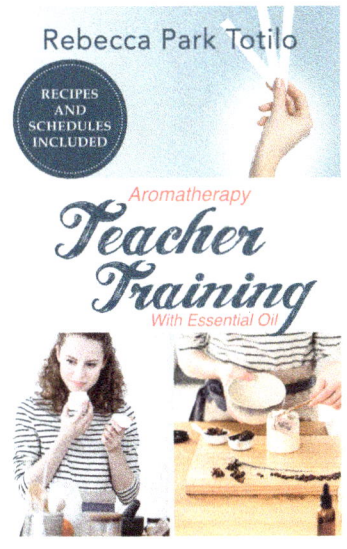

Aromatherapy Teacher Training With Essential Oil

Aromatherapy Teacher Training With Essential Oil provides the essential oil enthusiast the opportunity to craft and hone effective teaching methods for facilitating essential oils classes. This informative book will help you brainstorm and develop unique and interesting aromatherapy workshops, class outlines, and, most importantly, hands-on activities that will keep your students involved and wanting more! Using Rebecca Park Totilo's personal inspirational approach to aromatherapy training, you will come away with the knowledge and confidence to lead and teach your own short workshop or aromatherapy class. Inside this instructional book, you will find:

- The Science of Teaching - Learn how to teach different learning styles, discover your teaching methodology, and develop your own personal techniques for sharing about essential oils.
- The Class - Create a lesson plan from the many themes, choose the best oils to teach, and plan your class with icebreakers, blending projects, venues, and much more.
- Teaching Aromatherapy - Discover how to introduce the safe use of essential oils with detailed step-by-step instructions on demonstrating numerous types of blending projects.
- The Business of Teaching Aromatherapy - Have confidence in knowing what to charge for your classes, develop an elevator speech, and effective marketing for your course.
- Resources - Sample outline and timelines, basic recipes, and a glossary of terms are all included.

Sleep Better With Essential Oil

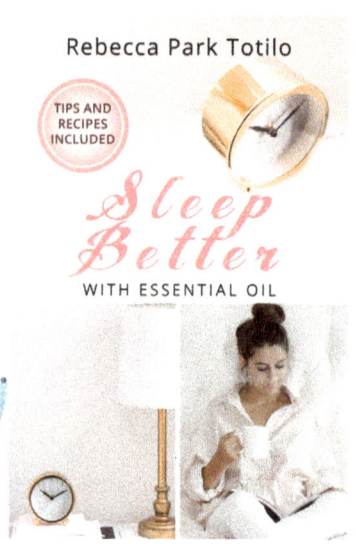

It can be hard to get optimal sleep in this modern age. Some people have trouble sleeping through the night because of things like a crying baby or a toddler who won't go to bed. For others, a busy work schedule and constant notifications on their phone can be distractions. And for some people, there's also the problem of having too much technology available. Social media and TV shows can be so distracting that they make it hard to get enough sleep. Even something as small and seemingly insignificant as drinking caffeine during the day or having a lumpy mattress can prevent restful sleep at night. What are we to do when distractions and outside forces steal our sleep?

Fortunately, there is hope for those struggling to get quality, consistent sleep. Hundreds of thousands of people worldwide have discovered the potent nature of essential oils to create a restful environment in their homes every night. The aroma of these oils can be combined with other healthy practices before bedtime for an even better experience. This book touches on some important aspects of sleeplessness and essential oils. Hopefully, it will answer questions you have on how to use essential oils at bedtime and create a more restful environment for getting the best sleep possible.

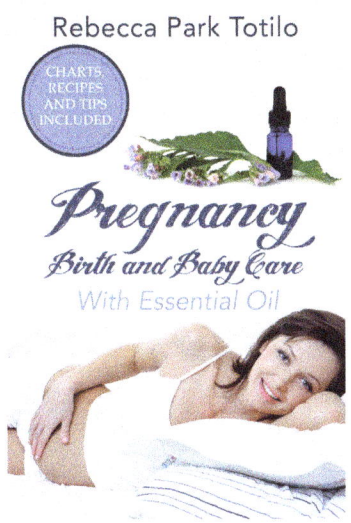

Pregnancy, Birth and Baby Care With Essential Oil

Pregnancy, Birth, and Baby Care With Essential Oil shows you how to safely use essential oils for all types of issues that arise during pregnancy, labor, and postpartum. Unlike traditional pregnancy guidebooks that follow conventional, fear-based instruction, this book offers a healthy approach to pregnancy, childbirth, and baby care, embracing a natural and safe way to use essential oils.

Full of advice and tips for a healthy pregnancy, Rebecca Park Totilo's researched-based remedies for common and troublesome symptoms guide you with the utmost care given to the health of you and your unborn child.

- Safe and Effective Essential Oils Treatments that address a range of ailments and concerns before and after the baby arrives. Details over 50 different pregnancy discomforts and challenges from morning sickness to insomnia, acne to backaches, heartburn to stretchmarks - and how aromatherapy can help.
- Numerous Charts outline specific essential oils safe for use during pregnancy, labor and delivery, nursing, and newborn care
- Detailed Profiles of 45 Essential Oils provides a comprehensive understanding of the medicinal properties, chemical makeup, and precautions of each essential oil.
- Over 100+ Essential Oils Recipes professionally formulated with step by step instructions for use in the bath, in a massage, and for diffusing around your home.

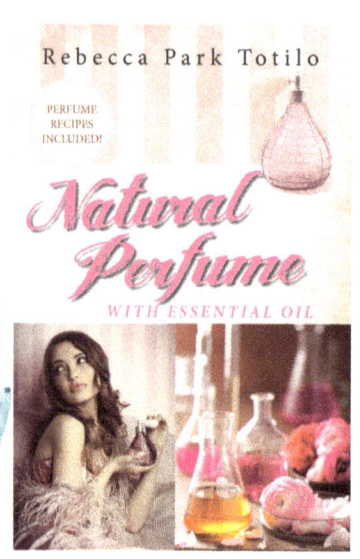

Natural Perfume With Essential Oil

Using the same classic perfumery techniques and processes as mainstream houses, a natural perfumer can blend, dilute, age and bottle his or her own signature scent, rivaling any name brand. Perfumes, body splashes, and colognes can be healthy too when created with pure essential oils and absolutes derived from botanical ingredients harvested from the earth. Natural perfumes can be eco-friendly, unlike their lab-created synthetic counterparts whose chemicals are considered toxic environmental hazards. Now you can create natural fragrances that are subtle, giving you an aura of sweet bliss within your breathing space—only a few feet from your body. When you leave the room, your fragrance goes with you. In this guide, you will discover how to create natural Eau de parfums that develop in layers, changing gradually with the chemistry of your skin. Working in unison with your body's chemistry, your fragrance gently evolves into your own signature scent, so you smell like you, not like everybody else. Discover how to create unique fragrances unlike anything on the market that will captivate your senses.

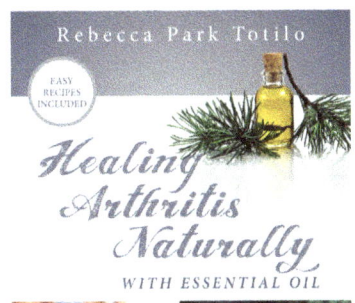

Healing Arthritis Naturally With Essential Oil

If you feel a bit like the tin man in the Wizard of Oz because your joints creak or don't move when you want them to, maybe they are asking you for oil - essential oils that is. Why live with pain or limited mobility if you don't have to? Medical research provides compelling evidence that essential oils can relieve pain and inflammation whether its due to a sports injury or arthritis, and offers the least invasive orthopedic treatment available. As the leading cause of disability in America today and the most common chronic disease to affect those over the age of 40, arthritis comes in over 100 different forms, and all share one main characteristic: joint inflammation. If you're one of the 50 million worldwide affected by arthritis, nature has provided a remedy. In this book, author Rebecca Park Totilo shares valuable information on the causes and symptoms of arthritis and how to use essential oils as a natural alternative. Discover which essential oils reduce inflammation and pain and how to formulate blends using essential oils. You will find dozens of recipes for lotions, salves, bath salts, and more in this how-to guide!

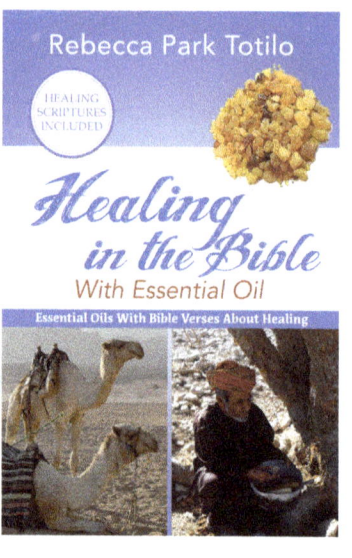

Healing In The Bible With Essential Oil

Since the creation, essential oils have been inhaled, applied to the body, and taken internally in which the benefits extended to every aspect of their being. Buried within the passages of scriptures lies a hidden treasure - possibly every man's answer to illness and disease. Now you can learn their secrets and discover how to transform your life and walk in divine health. In this book, Healing in the Bible With Essential Oil, Certified Aromatherapist Rebecca Park Totilo reveals various aspects of every fragrance mentioned in the Bible.

You will discover each essential oil:

- Rich biblical history and/or pagan roots
- Spiritual significance, symbolism, and hidden meaning
- Healing properties, including traditional uses, medicinal properties, and applications
- Scripture references, Hebrew or Greek meanings, and usage
- Rituals and recipes for making holy water, anointing oil, healing salves, and incense

Based on science and research, over 30 essential oil datasheets are included showing the breakdown of the chemical components, helping you to identify the oil's therapeutic benefits with safety information.

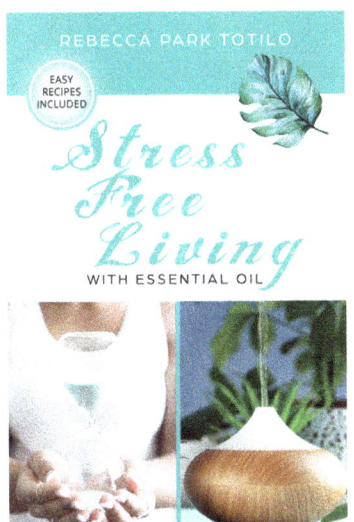

Stress-Free Living With Essential Oil

Everyone experiences stress from time to time. But when stress goes unchecked over time, it can play havoc on a person's health. Chronic stress results in a complete breakdown of the body and mental health. In Stress-Free Living With Essential Oil, author Rebecca Park Totilo offers a natural solution for handling the symptoms of stress using essential oils.

Based on scientific studies, Rebecca lists which essential oils can effectively reprogram the stress response on a chemical level in the brain and interrupt unhealthy stress responses - quickly shifting the body towards homeostasis. Discover how to live a stress-free life using essential oils. Numerous recipes and tips are included in this how-to guide!

www.ingramcontent.com/pod-product-compliance
Lightning Source LLC
Chambersburg PA
CBHW042128160426
43198CB00021B/2941